How to Prepare the Endometrium to Maximize Implantation Rates and IVF Success

T0179575

How to Prepare the Endometrium to Maximize Implantation Rates and IVF Success

Edited by
Gabor Kovacs
Monash University Victoria, Australia

Lois Salamonsen
Hudson Institute of Medical Research, Monash University Victoria, Australia

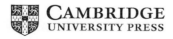

CAMBRIDGE
UNIVERSITY PRESS

University Printing House, Cambridge CB2 8BS, United Kingdom

One Liberty Plaza, 20th Floor, New York, NY 10006, USA

477 Williamstown Road, Port Melbourne, VIC 3207, Australia

314–321, 3rd Floor, Plot 3, Splendor Forum, Jasola District Centre, New Delhi – 110025, India

79 Anson Road, #06–04/06, Singapore 079906

Cambridge University Press is part of the University of Cambridge.

It furthers the University's mission by disseminating knowledge in the pursuit of
education, learning, and research at the highest international levels of excellence.

www.cambridge.org
Information on this title: www.cambridge.org/9781108402811
DOI: 10.1017/9781108236263

© Cambridge University Press 2019

First published 2019

Printed in the United Kingdom by TJ International Ltd. Padstow Cornwall

A catalogue record for this publication is available from the British Library.

Library of Congress Cataloging-in-Publication Data
Names: Kovacs, Gabor, 1947 April 6– editor. | Salamonsen, L. A. (Lois Adrienne), editor.
Title: How to prepare the endometrium to maximize implantation rates and IVF success / edited by Gabor
Kovacs, Lois Salamonsen.
Description: Cambridge, United Kingdom ; New York, NY: Cambridge University Press, 2019. | Includes
bibliographical references and index.
Identifiers: LCCN 2018027148 | ISBN 9781108402811
Subjects: | MESH: Embryo Transfer – methods | Endometrium – physiology | Fertilization in Vitro | Embryo
Implantation
Classification: LCC RG135 | NLM WQ 208 | DDC 618.1/780599–dc23
LC record available at https://lccn.loc.gov/2018027148

ISBN 978-1-108-40281-1 Paperback

Contents

Contributors

Siladitya Bhattacharya, MD, FRCOG
Institute of Applied Health Sciences, School of Medicine and Dentistry, University of Aberdeen, Scotland, UK

Giuseppe Botta, MD
Clinica C.G. Ruesch and Ospedale San Paolo, Naples, Italy

Annabelle Brennan, MBBS/LLB (Hons)
The Royal Women's Hospital, Melbourne, Victoria, Australia

Jan J. Brosens, MD, PhD, FRCOG
Division of Biomedical Sciences, Warwick Medical School, University Hospital, Warwickshire, UK
Tommy's National Miscarriage Research Centre, Warwick Medical School, University Hospital, Warwickshire, UK

Rohan Chodankar, MBBS, MD, MRCOG
MRC Centre for Reproductive Health, University of Edinburgh, UK

Ole Bjarne Christiansen, DMSc
Department of Obstetrics and Gynaecology, Aalborg University Hospital, Aalborg, Denmark
Recurrent Pregnancy Loss Clinic, Rigshospitalet, Copenhagen University Hospital, Copenhagen, Denmark

Patricia Díaz-Gimeno, PhD
Fundación Instituto Valenciano de Infertilidad (FIVI),
Instituto Universitario IVI (IUIVI)
Valencia University/INCLIVA, Spain

Eva Dimitriadis, PhD
Department of Obstetrics and Gynaecology, University of Melbourne, Australia

Tracey A. Edgell, BSc(Hons), PhD
Hudson Institute of Medical Research, Victoria, Australia

Jemma Evans, PhD
The Hudson Institute of Medical Research, Victoria, Australia

Juan A. Garcia-Velasco, MD, PhD
IVI Madrid, Madrid, Spain
Rey Juan Carlos University, Madrid, Spain

Gedis Grudzinskas, FRCOG
Consultant in Reproductive Medicine, London, UK

Natalie Hannan, PhD
Department of Obstetrics and Gynaecology, University of Melbourne, Melbourne, Australia

Martha Hickey, BA (Hons), MSc, MBChB, FRCOG, FRANZCOG, MD
Professor of Obstetrics, The University of Melbourne and the Royal Women's Hospital, Victoria, Australia

Andrew Horne, MB, ChB, PhD, FRCOG, FRCP Edin
MRC Centre for Reproductive Health, University of Edinburgh, UK

Tia Hunjan, MBChB, BSc
Queen Charlotte's and Chelsea Hospital, London, UK

Sarah Hunt, MBBS, FRANZCOG, MRM
Monash Health, Monash University and Monash IVF
Monash Medical Centre, Victoria, Australia

Jason Kasraie, BSc(Hons), MSc, DipRCPath
The Shropshire and Mid-Wales Fertility Centre, The Shrewsbury and Telford Hospitals NHS Trust, Shropshire, UK

Shirin Khanjani, MD, PhD, MRCOG
Imperial College, London, UK

Stuart Lavery, MRCOG, MSc, MBBCh
Department of Reproductive Medicine, Imperial College, London, UK

Ashley Moffett, MD, MRCP, MRCPath, FRCOG
University of Cambridge, Cambridge, UK

Inmaculada Moreno, PhD
Department Research and Development, Igenomix Spain, Valencia, Spain
Department of Obstetrics and Gynecology, Stanford University, Stanford, CA, USA

Luciano G. Nardo, MD, MRCOG
Reproductive Health Group, Centre for Reproductive Health, Cheshire, UK

Guiying Nie, PhD
Centre for Reproductive Health, Hudson Institute of Medical Research, Victoria, Australia

Kathinka Marie Nyborg, MD
Recurrent Pregnancy Loss Clinic, Rigshospitalet, Copenhagen University Hospital, Copenhagen, Denmark

Yuval Or, MD
Reproductive Medicine and IVF Unit, Kaplan Medical Center, Rehovot, Israel

Nikoletta Panagiotopoulou, MRCOG, MSc
Aberdeen Centre for Reproductive Medicine, Aberdeen, Scotland, UK

Terhi T. Piltonen, MD, PhD
Finnish Medical Foundation, Department of Obstetrics and Gynecology, PEDEGO

Research Unit, Medical Research Center, Oulu University Hospital, University of Oulu, Finland

Sarah A. Robertson, PhD
Robinson Research Institute and Adelaide Medical School, University of Adelaide, South Australia, Australia

Tarique Salman, MBChB, MRCOG
Reproductive Health Group, Centre for Reproductive Health, Cheshire, UK

Gamal I. Serour, FRCOG, FRCS
International Islamic Center for Population Studies and Research, Al Azhar University, Cairo, Egypt

Khaldoun Sharif, MBBCh, MD, MFFP, FRCOG, FACOG
Jordan Hospital, Amman, Jordan

David J. Sharkey, PhD
Robinson Research Institute and Adelaide Medical School, University of Adelaide, South Australia, Australia

Zeev Shoham, MD
Director of the Fertility and IVF Unit Kaplan Medical Center, Rehovot Israel Affiliated to the Hadassah Medical Center, The Hebrew University, Jerusalem, Israel

Dr Norman Shreeve, BM, BSc
Wellcome Trust PhD for Clinicians Programme, University of Cambridge, Cambridge, UK
Addenbrooke's Hospital, Cambridge, UK

Carlos Simon, MD, PhD
Igenomix Spain, Valencia, Spain
Department of Obstetrics and Gynecology, Stanford University, Stanford, CA, USA
Department of Obstetrics and Gynecology, University of Valencia/INCLIVA, Valencia, Spain

Department of Obstetrics and Gynecology, Baylor College of Medicine, Houston, TX, USA

Jamie Stanhiser, MD
Division of Reproductive Endocrinology and Infertility, University of North Carolina, Chapel Hill, NC, USA

Shreeya Tewary, MB ChB MRCOG
Division of Biomedical Sciences, Warwick Medical School, University Hospital, Warwickshire, UK

Beverley Vollenhoven, PhD, FRANZCOG, CREI
Department of Obstetrics and Gynaecology, Monash University, Monash Health and Monash IVF, Victoria, Australia

Steven L. Young MD, PhD
Professor, Reproductive Endocrinology & Infertility, Obstetrics & Gynecology, Cell Biology and Physiology, University of North Carolina School of Medicine, Chapel Hill, NC, USA

Preface

The embryo transfer is the final step in the in vitro fertilization (IVF) treatment cycle, and it is the step with the greatest failure rate. Success requires implantation which depends on the normality of the embryo its ability to achieve apposition, adhesion and attachment. For this to occur successfully, endometrium has to be receptive. Endometrial receptivity is considered the 'Black Box' of reproductive technologies. While considerable advances have been made in obtaining oocytes, fertilization and embryo development in vitro, little progress has been achieved in improving implantation rates following transfer of a high-quality embryo. This will require a greater understanding of how the endometrium becomes receptive, the blastocyst–maternal interactions during the final stages of blastocyst development in the microenvironment within the uterine cavity, and how appropriate preparation of both the endometrial epithelium and the developing decidua are critical to establish a viable pregnancy. The contributions in this volume, from well-recognized experts in their fields, will update clinicians and scientists alike on the latest developments in the field.

Chapter 1

Physiology of Endometrial Development through the Cycle and Implantation

Annabelle Brennan and Martha Hickey

1.1 Introduction

The monthly female reproductive cycle involves a pattern of cyclic sex steroid changes to prepare the endometrium for potential implantation of an embryo. This chapter outlines the physiological aspects of the reproductive cycle, including the production of gonado-trophic hormones, their relationship to the ovarian hormones, the development of follicles, release of the ovum and either potential implantation of the blastocyst or menstruation in the absence of pregnancy.

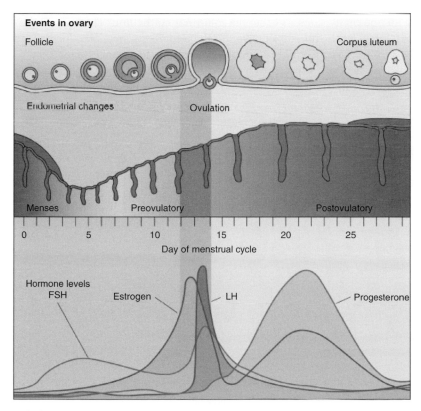

Figure 1.1 The female reproductive cycle – the follicular, endometrial and hormonal changes throughout the cycle are demonstrated
Source: Gartner, LP. *Textbook of Histology*, Fourth Edition. Chapter 20, Female Reproductive System (Elsevier, 2017).

The endometrial cycle has two distinct phases, each with different functions required of the tissue. This chapter utilises these endometrial phases as a framework to examine the reproductive cycle as a whole.

The preovulatory, or follicular, phase is a two-week period involving the development of the ovarian follicles usually resulting in ovulation. This phase is oestrogen dominant, repairing and priming a new endometrial layer after the previous menstruation.

The luteal phase is the two-week period following ovulation. This progesterone-dominant phase matures the endometrium, providing a nutritious site for potential implantation. In the absence of pregnancy, after withdrawal of hormones, the now-thickened endometrium is shed during menstruation and the cycle can commence again.

1.2 Endometrial Structure

The endometrium consists of three layers. The basal layer resting above the myometrium is the stratum basalis. The stratum compactum and stratum spongiosum lie above the basalis and together form the stratum functionalis. The functionalis layer undergoes cyclical change in response to hormone fluctuations and is shed with menstruation, leaving the stratum basalis to regenerate a new functionalis the following cycle. These layers are demonstrated in Figure 1.2.

Several cell types are contained within the endometrium. The most superficial layer, lining the uterine cavity, consists of simple columnar epithelium. Throughout the endometrium this luminal epithelium dips down into the underlying stroma to form glands, whose secretory function is intrinsically reliant on the monthly hormonal cycle.

The vascular network supplying the endometrium involves a sophisticated plexus of vessels with varying hormonal sensitivities. The uterine arteries branching from the internal

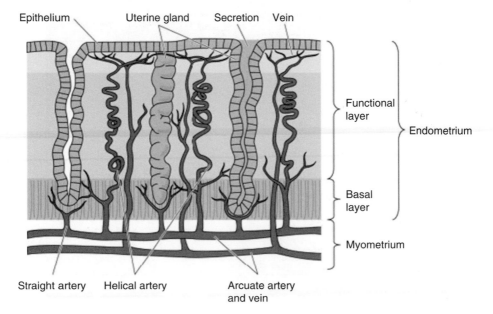

Figure 1.2 Endometrial histology – the basal and functional layers of the endometrium are demonstrated with the underlying vascular supply
Source: Gartner, LP. *Textbook of Histology*, Fourth Edition. Chapter 20, Female Reproductive System (Elsevier, 2017).

iliac vessels give rise to the radial arteries, which supply the underlying myometrium. These vessels branch into straight arterioles supplying the stratum basalis and coiled spiral, or helical, arterioles supplying the more superficial stratum functionalis. Blood from the sub-epithelial capillaries then drains into a venous plexus that mirrors the arterial supply. The vascular supply to the endometrium is demonstrated in Figure 1.2.

The basal vessels are surrounded by smooth muscle and are not influenced by cyclic sex steroid variation. However, the more superficial vessels consist mainly of endothelium. Without the surrounding smooth muscle support, these vessels are more easily influenced by endothelial growth factors, hormonal fluctuations, hypoxia and mechanical stress [1].

1.3 Follicular Phase

The hypothalamic-pituitary-gonadal axis regulates ovarian sex steroid production that leads to regular shedding of the superficial endometrium and blood loss when pregnancy does not occur. Release of hypothalamic gonadotropin-releasing hormone (GnRH) occurs in a rhythmic pulsatile pattern, approximately every one to two hours [2]. GnRH is trans-ported to the anterior pituitary gland via a complex capillary bed, the hypothalamic-hypophyseal portal blood system. In response to the effect of GnRH, the anterior pituitary produces two hormones, follicle-stimulating hormone (FSH) and luteinizing hor-mone (LH).

The prepubertal ovary contains a large collection of oocytes, each surrounded by a layer of granulosa cells and referred to as primordial follicles. With the onset of puberty, the increasing role of FSH and LH causes oocyte growth as well as the formation of additional layers of granulosa cells; the follicles are now termed 'primary follicles'. It is these primary follicles that undergo maturation and potential ovulation during the monthly ovarian cycle.

At the start of the follicular phase, FSH released from the anterior pituitary causes rapid growth of the granulosa cell layer in several primary follicles. A layer of thecal cells forms around the granulosa cell mass encapsulating the follicle.

Granulosa cells produce several hormones, including oestrogen, and rapid follicular growth results in increasing oestrogen levels. Oestrogen release then stimulates develop-ment of more FSH and LH receptors, increasing the cells' sensitivity to the hormones and triggering further proliferation of both granulosa and thecal cell layers. Meanwhile, LH stimulates thecal production of androstenedione, which the granulosa cells assist in con-verting to oestrogen, further contributing to the rapid rise in oestrogen levels.

Prior to ovulation, one follicle begins to grow more rapidly than the others (dominant or leading follicle), potentially due to increased receptor expression and thus sensitivity to FSH [3]. Within the dominant follicle, the oestrogen-containing follicular fluid secreted by the granulosa cells accumulates in a sac referred to as the follicular antrum. The increasing oestrogen production acts as negative feedback to the anterior pituitary to reduce the production of both FSH and LH, which accounts for the dips in gonadotrophic hormone production (Figure 1.1). The withdrawal of gonadotrophic stimulation causes the remain-ing follicles to undergo atresia, while the intrinsic oestrogen from the dominant follicle is sufficient for its ongoing growth.

However, when oestrogen production from the dominant follicle reaches peak levels, it contrastingly acts as positive feedback to the anterior pituitary, stimulating a sudden surge in LH and, to a lesser extent, FSH production. Meanwhile, the increasing LH levels stimulate the granulosa cells to produce two other sex steroids, progesterone and inhibin. Inhibin reduces production of FSH from the anterior pituitary, accounting for the lower peak of FSH compared to LH observed (Figure 1.1).

The high levels of LH and increasing production of progesterone reduce the secretion of oestrogen and stimulate ovulation. Follicular angiogenesis and prostaglandin release cause swelling of the follicle. Simultaneous release of enzymes from thecal cells begins to weaken the follicle capsule, until it eventually ruptures, releasing the ovum. In a normal 28-day cycle, this process occurs at day 14.

1.3.1 Follicular Phase Endometrium

Following menstruation signalling the end of the previous cycle, the endometrial layer is thin. The endometrium must repair before the next ovulation to provide opportunity for implantation. The follicular phase involves proliferation of both stromal and glandular layers of the endometrium with accompanying angiogenesis.

It appears that endometrial vascular cells contain both oestrogen and progesterone receptors [4]. However, the initial repair of the endometrium commences shortly after the onset of menstruation, when the circulating ovarian hormone levels remain low. This would suggest that local factors, including angiogenic growth factors and prostaglandins, are essential to endometrial repair. Interestingly, many of these factors are released in the pro-inflammatory and intermittently hypoxic environment of the late luteal phase prior to menstruation. This suggests that progesterone withdrawal is not only an important trigger of menstruation but also indirectly relevant to the subsequent repair of endometrial tissue [5].

The growth factors and chemical mediators present in the tissue work to re-epithelialise the endometrium in a number of days. Angiogenesis and vascular permeability are vital in ensuring adequate delivery of nutrients to the newly forming endometrium. In addition, increasing oestrogen levels cause proliferation and growth of the stromal and glandular cells. However, the secretory function of the endometrial glands does not mature without the presence of progesterone during the luteal phase.

The aim of the oestrogen-dominant follicular phase is to repair the previously shed stratum functionalis. A thickened, oedematous endometrium is formed in preparation for ovulation and potential implantation.

1.4 Luteal Phase

Following the release of the ovum during ovulation, the follicle contains the remnant granulosa and theca cells. Under the influence of the high levels of LH at this time, these cells undergo a process of luteinisation involving cholesterol deposition vital for steroidogenesis. The cells are now referred to as lutein cells and the cell mass is termed the 'corpus luteum', meaning 'yellow body', referring to the characteristic yellow appearance of the cells caused by intracellular cholesterol.

The primary hormonal focus of the follicular phase is the rising oestrogen levels, which prime the endometrium and initiate the essential preovulatory LH surge. During the late follicular phase, LH alters the function of the granulosa cells, changing the hormonal environment to one of mainly progesterone secretion. This effect continues during the luteal phase, with the corpus luteum producing increasing amounts of progesterone and, to a lesser extent, oestrogen. This change in sex steroid production can be observed in Figure 1.1.

The importance of progesterone during the luteal phase lies in maturation of the endometrium. Progesterone enhances development of the endometrial glands and initiates secretions. It stimulates angiogenesis with the formation of tight, coiled vessels, which become full and permeable, creating oedema within the endometrial stroma. These characteristic histological findings of the luteal-phase endometrium reflect the nutrient-rich, thickened endometrium prepared for potential implantation of the fertilised ovum.

During the luteal phase, elevated levels of progesterone and oestrogen released from the corpus luteum act as negative feedback on the anterior pituitary to minimise secretion of FSH and LH. Furthermore, the release of inhibin from the lutein cells further suppresses gonadotrophin secretion, mainly FSH.

However, the withdrawal of gonadotrophic stimulation eventually causes degeneration of the corpus luteum. As the cells atrophy and the cell mass degenerates, the production of progesterone and oestrogen dwindles, removing the negative feedback effect on the anterior pituitary stimulating the release of both FSH and LH.

1.4.1 Luteal Phase Endometrium

During the mid-luteal phase, the progesterone-dominant environment is one focused on haemostasis. The hormone encourages a stable endometrium for blastocyst implantation, protecting against haemorrhage that could compromise the success of the pregnancy.

Haemostasis is encouraged via several mechanisms. Following the oestrogen-stimulated rapid growth of the endometrium during the proliferative phase, progesterone acts to limit uncontrolled angiogenesis. It also stimulates the release of tissue factor, a high-affinity receptor for factor VII, playing a vital role in the initiation of the clotting cascade [6].

Progesterone is also involved in the inhibition of matrix metalloproteinases (MMP). MMP are enzymes responsible for the degradation of the structural extracellular matrix. They are largely released from the endometrial stromal cells and, to a lesser extent, endometrial leucocytes [7,8,9,10]. The inhibition of MMP expression stabilises the endometrial stroma and the underlying vascular network, preventing haemorrhage.

By the late luteal phase, the stromal cells are the only endometrial cellular component with progesterone receptors [9]. In the absence of pregnancy, degeneration of the corpus luteum and progesterone withdrawal therefore removes the stabilising effect of progesterone on the cells of the perivascular stroma. Progesterone withdrawal allows the perivascular stromal cells to produce pro-inflammatory chemokines, including prostaglandins, interleukins and tumour necrosis factor-α, which stimulate vascular permeability and attract endometrial leucocytes, including neutrophils, macrophages and mast cells.

Furthermore, progesterone withdrawal likely stimulates a period of vasospasm through its effect on the perivascular stroma; vasoconstriction and tissue hypoxia are followed by vasodilation and subsequent reperfusion injury [11]. This environment up-regulates the pro-inflammatory state with further release of inflammatory chemical mediators and their cellular recruits.

Proliferation of leucocytes occurs within the endometrium as well as migration from the peripheral circulation [8]. The subsequent release of lytic enzymes and MMP destabilises the endometrial matrix. In particular, degradation of the perivascular matrix causes weakening and disruption to the vasculature and results in haemorrhage. The vascular fragility and propensity to bleed are exacerbated by the concomitant oestrogen withdrawal of the late luteal phase [12]. Furthermore, proteolytic destruction of the remaining stromal matrix causes cellular breakdown and tissue sloughing.

These changes are accompanied by the loss of other progesterone-based haemostatic measures. Hormone withdrawal reduces the expression of coagulant factors, including tissue factor and plasminogen activator inhibitor-l, and impairs platelet function [13,14]. There is additional up-regulation of anticoagulant factors such as tissue plasminogen activator and urokinase. The result is a haemorrhagic environment favouring tissue destruction. The presence of desquamated cells and the associated chemical mediators triggers uterine contractility to promote expulsion of the tissue.

1.5 Implantation

Following fertilisation of the ovum, successful implantation requires a viable blastocyst to communicate effectively with a receptive endometrium, which can support the growing embryo until the placenta is able to supply adequate nutrition. The endometrium is considered receptive for a relatively short period of time each cycle, likely several days. This period is referred to as the 'window of implantation', beyond which the blastocyst cannot adhere and menstruation results [15,16].

The initial communication between the developing blastocyst and the endometrium is mediated by a range of factors secreted by the epithelial cells, guiding the orientation and attachment of the blastocyst. The complex role and interaction of these factors are discussed elsewhere in this book.

The luminal epithelium of the endometrium forms projections termed 'pinopodes', which assist in the adhesion of the blastocyst to the endometrial lining [17]. Once attached, the trophoblast cells strongly adhere to the epithelium and release a range of lytic enzymes allowing invasion of the blastocyst into the deeper endometrial stroma and absorption of nutrients [18,19].

The blastocyst is surrounded by a layer of cells, trophoblasts. Implantation is associated with proliferation of the trophoblasts into two distinct layers. The cytotrophoblasts form the inner layer and fuse to form an outer layer of multinucleated cells termed 'syncitiotrophoblasts'.

In the absence of pregnancy, the degeneration of the corpus luteum causes progesterone withdrawal, resulting in menstruation and a new reproductive cycle. A successful pregnancy therefore requires that the endometrial tissue has sufficient exposure to progesterone to stabilise the endometrial lining and prevent expulsion of the trophoblast.

Consequently, the syncitiotrophoblast cells secrete human chorionic gonadotrophin (HCG), a hormone structurally and functionally similar to LH. HCG thereby maintains the corpus luteum, allowing continued production of progesterone. The importance of progesterone at this point lies in the development of a supportive endometrium and prevention of uterine contractility that could expel the implanting blastocyst. The corpus luteum is the main source of progesterone and oestrogens for the developing pregnancy for the first two to three months, beyond which the placenta provides sufficient hormone production to maintain the pregnancy and the corpus luteum involutes.

The process of blastocyst invasion in the progesterone-dominant environment triggers the decidualisation of the endometrium. The formation of the decidua is a process of stromal cell growth and intracellular accumulation of nutrients, activation of the glandular secretory function and angiogenesis to support the developing blastocyst.

During invasion, the syncitiotrophoblasts form villous projections into the stroma. Until blood flow develops, the blastocyst is maintained by absorption of nutrients across the villi from the glandular secretions and decidual cells [19]. Blastocyst invasion and decidualisation then trigger the release of various angiogenic factors. This process stimulates angiogenesis of fetal vessels and vascular remodelling of the maternal uterine spiral arterioles by invasive trophoblasts to form feto-maternal circulatory connections allowing diffusion of nutrients and waste [20,21,22,23,24].

Invasion of maternal vessels by trophoblasts creates obvious potential for haemorrhage compromising implantation and placentation. The decidual cells play an important role in maintaining haemostasis via increased production of tissue factor and plasminogen activator inhibitor-l. These haemostatic mediators promote thrombin formation and prevent fibrinolysis, creating an anticoagulant environment [14].

The endometrium appears to play an active role in blastocyst selection, rather than passively accepting the attaching embryo. Abnormal embryos trigger a chemically mediated signal within the endometrium. Following the process of decidualisation, the stromal cells appear to have the ability to respond to these signals by engulfing the blastocyst and inhibiting the release of biochemical implantation factors, ultimately causing expulsion of the blastocyst with endometrial bleeding. Consequently, it is suggested that inadequate decidualisation results in loss of embryo selection and may be implicated in early or recurrent pregnancy loss [25,26].

1.6 Conclusion

The monthly female reproductive cycle involves a complex cascade of hormones to allow ovulation, fertilisation and potential implantation of a blastocyst. The multilayer structure of the endometrium is intrinsic to its cyclical function. Each month the superficial layers are primed for potential implantation and then, in the absence of pregnancy, shed and renewed to allow the cycle to commence again.

Many of the processes involved in this cycle are triggered directly by rhythmical hormonal fluctuations, relying on either hormonal stimulation or withdrawal to occur. The development of the ovum, ovulation and maturation of the endometrium are all examples. There are also some aspects that are indirectly related to hormone function through the flow-on effects of intermediate messengers. The premenstrual inflammatory tissue response and the initial repair of the endometrium are examples where tissue changes are indirectly influenced by hormones via the release of local chemical mediators.

The physiological principles behind the monthly reproductive cycle have long been understood. Yet increasing knowledge of the complexity of chemical pathways, including molecular and genetic involvement, has assisted in identifying possible contributors to infertility and early pregnancy loss. The result has been a greater understanding of potential areas for medical intervention.

References

1. Mathur R et al. Endometrial Angiogenesis: Physiology and Clinical Implications. *The Journal of Family Planning and Reproductive Health Care* 2000; 28, 4: 173–174.

2. Hall J E, Guyton A C. *Guyton and Hall Textbook of Medical Physiology* 2011; p. 1020. Saunders Elsevier: Philadelphia.

3. Kumar P et al. Luteinizing Hormone and Its Dilemma in Ovulation Induction. *Journal of Human Reproductive Sciences* 2011; 4, 1: 2–7.

4. Rogers P A W and Gargett C E. The Vascular System in the Endometrium: Introduction and Overview. *Vascular Morphogenesis in the Female Reproductive System* 2001; p. 215. Birkhauser: Boston.

5. Maybin J A et al. Progesterone: A Pivotal Hormone at Menstruation. *Annals of the New York Academy of Sciences* 2011; 1221: 88–97.

6. Lockwood CJ. Mechanisms of Normal and Abnormal Endometrial Bleeding. *Menopause* 2011; 18, 4: 408–411.

7. Dong J et al. Matrix Metalloproteinases and Their Specific Tissue Inhibitors in Menstruation. *Reproduction* 2002; 123: 621–631.

8. Salamonsen L A et al. Regulation of Matrix Metalloproteinases in Human Endometrium. *Human Reproduction* 2000; 15, Suppl. 3: 112–119.

9. Salamonsen L A et al. Endometrial Leukocytes and Menstruation. *Human Reproduction* 2000: 6, 1: 16–27.

10. Salamonsen L A et al. Matrix Metalloproteinases in Normal Menstruation. *Human Reproduction* 1996; 11, Suppl. 2: 124–133.

11. Kelly R W et al. Cytokine Control in Human Endometrium. *Reproduction* 2001; 121: 3–19.

12. Clemetson C A et al. Capillary Strength and the Menstrual Cycle. *Annals of the New York Academy of Sciences* 1962; 93: 279–299.

13. Hickey M and Fraser I S. The Clinical Relevance of Disturbances of Uterine Vascular Growth, Remodeling and Repair. *Vascular Morphogenesis in the Female Reproductive System* 2001; p. 229. Birkhauser: Boston.

14. Lockwood C J et al. Decidual Cell Regulation of Haemostasis During Implantation and Menstruation. *Annals of the New York Academy of Sciences* 1997; 828: 188–193.

15. Tabibzadeh S. Implantation: From Basics to the Clinic. *Annals of the New York Academy of Sciences* 1997; 828: 131–136.

16. Singh M et al. Bridging Endometrial Receptivity and Implantation: Network of Hormones, Cytokines, and Growth Factors. *Journal of Endocrinology* 2011; 210: 5–14.

17. Lopata A et al. 'Pinopodes' and Implantation. *Reviews in Endocrine and Metabolic Disorders* 2002; 33: 77–86.

18. Diedrich K et al. The Role of Endometrium and Embryo in Human Implantation. *Human Reproduction* 2007; 13, 4: 365–377.

19. Salamonsen L A et al. The Microenvironment of Human Implantation: Determinants of Reproductive Success. *American Journal of Reproductive Immunology* 2016; 75: 218–225.

20. Hannan N J et al. Role of Chemokines in the Endometrium and in Embryo Implantation. *Current Opinions in Obstetrics and Gynaecology* 2007; 19: 266–272.

21. Bagheri A et al. Angiogenic Factors in Relation to Embryo Implantation. *International Journal of Reproduction, Contraception, Obstetrics and Gynaecology* 2014: 3, 4: 872–879.

22. Chwalisz K et al. Role of Nitric Oxide in Implantation and Menstruation. *Human Reproduction* 2000; 15, Suppl. 3: 96–111.

23. Torry DS et al. Angiogenesis in Implantation. *Journal of Assisted*

Reproduction and Genetics 2007: 24: 303–315.

24. Kilman H J. Uteroplacental Blood Flow: The Story of Decidualisation, Menstruation and Trophoblast Invasion. *American Journal of Pathology* 2000; 157, 6: 1759–1768.

25. Teklenburg G et al. Natural Selection of Human Embryos: Decidualizing Endometrial Stromal Cells Serve as Sensors of Embryo Quality upon Implantation. *PLoS ONE* 2010; 5, 4: 1–6.

26. Salker M et al. Natural Selection of Human Embryos: Impaired Decidualisation of Endometrium Disables Embryo-maternal Interactions and Causes Recurrent Pregnancy Loss. *PLoS ONE* 2010; 5, 4: 1–7.

Chapter 2

Molecular and Cellular Basis of Human Embryo Implantation

Guiying Nie and Eva Dimitriadis

2.1 Overview of Human Embryo Implantation Cascades

Embryo implantation in humans involves sequential steps of apposition, adhesion, and invasion of an implantation-competent blastocyst into a hormonally prepared receptive endometrium [1,2]. The embryo enters the uterine cavity approximately four days after ovulation; it then sheds the zona pellucida and apposes with its polar trophectoderm (the site near the inner cell mass (ICM)) to the endometrial luminal epithelium. The blastocyst is only loosely attached at this stage as it can be washed off. More firm adhesion occurs once the embryo has stably settled upon the endometrium. Thereafter, the entire embryo traverses between the epithelial cells, penetrates the basal lamina (the extracellular matrix on which the epithelium sits), and invades into the underlying stroma. The luminal epithelium then reseals over the implantation site, completely encapsulating the embryo within the tissue [1].

Human implantation is distinct in many respects from any other species. It is a complex yet highly coordinated and continuing process that involves intricate physical and molecular interaction between the embryo and the host endometrium. The embryo has to be well developed and capable of implantation. The endometrium also needs to transform into a receptive state for implantation to occur [3]. In each menstrual cycle, the endometrium is receptive to an embryo only for a temporal and limited period, which is known as the "window of implantation." This window begins at around seven days after the luteinizing hormone (LH) surge and remains open between approximately days 20 and 24 within a 28-day menstrual cycle. At other times the endometrium is non-receptive to embryo implantation. Ovarian hormones estrogen and progesterone are the master regulators of endometrial remodeling, and changing blood levels of these hormones orchestrate the establishment of endometrial receptivity in synchrony with blastocyst development for implantation [2].

2.2 Endometrial Epithelial Remodeling for Embryo Attachment

2.2.1 Epithelial Plasma Membrane Transformation

As the implanting embryo first interacts with the luminal epithelium of the endometrium, this part of the maternal tissue undergoes major remodeling to prepare for embryo attachment. The epithelial cells change shape from a columnar to a cuboidal type, and this morphological change is accompanied by substantial alterations in the plasma membrane, which are collectively referred to as the "plasma membrane transformation" [4]. One significant change is the conversion of the apical plasma membrane from containing long and regular microvilli to a flat and microvilli-poor surface [5]. Apical plasma membrane flattening is a common feature of receptivity development across many species, and this change allows a closer physical contact between the endometrium and the blastocyst. Furthermore, apical protrusions called uterodomes or pinopodes grow on the surface of these cells [6]; these structures are believed to absorb uterine fluid to immobilize the blastocyst to the endometrial surface.

In addition, the membrane–cytoskeleton interaction also changes substantially [4,5], involving reorganization and redistribution of the actin filaments. In the non-receptive state, the epithelial cell cytoplasm contains a prominent network of well-organized actin microfilaments (terminal web), providing a platform to which bundled actin filaments anchor the apical membrane microvilli and connect the membrane to the cytoplasm. At receptivity, the terminal web is lost, and the actin microfilaments are rearranged and dissociated from the membrane [4,5].

These structural alterations are achieved by considerable biochemical and molecular changes, one of which is the removal of cytoplasmic peripheral membrane protein ezrin from the apical membrane. Ezrin acts as an intermediate between the plasma membrane and the actin cytoskeleton; it tethers actin filaments to the plasma membrane and anchors membrane proteins at specific sites to maintain epithelial organization and cell surface structure. Loss of ezrin results in short, thick, and randomly oriented microvilli. Ezrin strongly binds to scaffolding protein EBP50, and this binding compartmentalizes ezrin to the apical membrane and enables it to interact with actin. Specifically, the C-terminal tail of EBP50 provides the key binding site for ezrin. Recent studies suggest that during endometrial conversion to receptivity, the C-terminal tail of EBP50 is enzymatically cleaved by proprotein convertase 6 (PC6), and this seemingly simple cleavage profoundly alters EBP50–ezrin interaction and the cytoskeleton–membrane connection [7].

2.2.2 Epithelial Glycocalyx Remodeling

The external surface of epithelial plasma membrane is covered by "glycocalyx," which is composed largely of heavily glycosylated mucins that form the gel-like layer. More than 46 large glycoproteins have been identified on the apical surface of human endometrial epithelium. A thick glycocalyx lubricates the epithelial surface and protects the cells from mechanical/chemical injury; it also provides a physical barrier to microbes. However, a thick glycocalyx hinders blastocyst attachment, and redistribution or thinning of glycocalyx is thus necessary for embryo implantation. Mucin-1, a large and heavily glycosylated transmembrane protein, represents a relatively well-studied endometrial epithelial mucin protein for implantation. In mice, endometrial epithelial glycocalyx thinning is signified by a dramatic reduction in mucin-1 through down-regulation of its mRNA at the transcription level [8], and failure of this down-regulation causes implantation failure. This is in accordance with the notion that mucin-1 poses a steric hindrance for blastocyst attachment. However, in women, mucin-1 level in endometrial epithelium is increased rather than decreased in the window of implantation [9], suggesting that the strategies of endometrial epithelial glycocalyx remodeling differ considerably between species.

This has led to the speculation that, in contrast to mice, glycocalyx alteration in the human endometrial epithelium may be regulated at the posttranscriptional and/or posttranslational level. Consistent with this, TACE/ADAM17-mediated cleavage of the ectodomain of mucin-1 has been proposed as a mechanism of reducing the glycocalyx thickness in the human endometrium for receptivity. However, it remains controversial whether ADAM17 is the sheddase responsible for mucin-1 removal, as ADAM17 expression is not always up-regulated in the window of implantation. On the other hand, in vitro studies show that mucin-1 is removed locally by blastocyst-derived factors at the site of human blastocyst attachment [10], indicating that in humans the implanting embryo actively directs endometrial epithelial glycocalyx remodeling for implantation.

Furthermore, posttranslational regulation of another large surface glycoprotein, dystroglycan (DG), has been linked to endometrial receptivity in women [11]. DG consists of α- and β-subunits; while α-DG anchors within the plasma membrane, α-DG localizes extracellularly through non-covalent attachment to α-DG. The central region of α-DG outside the cell is needed to mediate adhesion, but it is hidden and obstructed by its large N-terminus (α-DG-N). The full-length α-DG in the human endometrial epithelium is thus a barrier for embryo attachment [11]. It is shown that PC6 proteolytically removes α-DG-N specifically in the receptive phase, exposing the central α-DG and transforming DG from a barrier to an adhesive molecule on the epithelial surface [11]. These studies highlight the importance of posttranslational control, particularly by proteases, in the regulation of human endometrial epithelial glycocalyx remodeling for receptivity.

2.2.3   Epithelial Ion Channel Activation

Ion channels are a group of transmembrane proteins that allow ions to flow across cell or organelle membranes. These channels, via controlling ion flow and ion gradients, regulate many cellular processes such as neuronal signal transmission, muscle contraction, epithelial secretion and fluid absorption, as well as cell proliferation and apoptosis [12]. These channels are tightly regulated by hormones as well as mechanical forces, temperature, and chemical substances.

At least 14 types of ion channels, including the Na^+, Cl^-, K^+, and $Ca2^+$ channels, have been identified in the endometrium and shown to play an important role in regulating receptivity for implantation [12]. One major mechanism of this regulation is through controlling uterine fluid, which reduces dramatically from ~110–180 ul to ~5–35 ul when the endometrium enters the receptive phase [12]. In addition, the electrolyte concentrations of the fluid also change significantly; for instance, the sodium ions decrease whereas the potassium ions increase [12]. These remarkable changes suggest that the luminal epithelium actively absorbs fluid during this time – a significant impact of which is to minimize blastocyst movement; this is believed to be critical because the blastocyst is very small (<0.2 mm in diameter in humans) relative to the uterine cavity [12], and a stable contact can be established only if the embryo is not freely moving. The importance of uterine fluid control for implantation has been well proven in assisted reproductive technology (ART) clinics, and in current practice the volume of fluid to be transferred with the embryo is limited to 20–60 µl to maximize implantation. Conversely, excessive uterine fluid buildup because of hydrosalpinges is strongly linked to implantation failure in ART cycles. Apart from fluid regulation, ion channels are also shown to indirectly regulate the expression of many implantation-associated genes, by controlling signaling pathways to activate or inactivate certain transcription factors [12].

2.3 Endometrial Stromal Cell Decidualization

Human endometrial stromal cells begin to differentiate (decidualize) around day 23 of each menstrual cycle regardless of the presence of a blastocyst. It involves transformation of the elongated fibroblast-like stromal cells into larger and rounded secretory decidual cells. If implantation occurs, decidualization proceeds, forming the decidual cells of pregnancy [13]. Progesterone is the main physiological stimulus of decidualization, while it is also clear that liganded or unliganded progesterone receptor and the cAMP/PKA pathway are also absolutely required for decidualization. Recent evidence demonstrates that other steroid receptors (ER, GR, MR, and AR) have unique roles in decidualization and in the interplay between the different steroid receptors. Progesterone activates both PR and MR and may drive decidualization at least partly via its actions on these receptors.

There is abundant evidence that locally produced factors progress progesterone-induced decidualization. Such local regulators include cytokines and proteases [14]. Decidualization begins in endometrial stromal cells surrounding the spiral arterioles, and it is also likely that vascular cell factors such as VEGF-D contribute to decidualization. Recent studies reveal important roles for epigenetic regulators and noncoding RNA in the progression of decidualization. Other cell types in the endometrium area are also likely to regulate decidualization, although these have not been extensively studied. It is not known if glandular epithelial cells secrete factors basally to regulate decidualization. It is likely to be the case, although there is little evidence in humans. Endometrial leukocytes, including uterine-specific NK, mast, T cells, and dendritic cells, are critical for mediating decidual angiogenesis during the initiation of pregnancy; it is not known whether they also drive decidualization in the peri-implantation period. However, decidualized stromal cells can influence the function and differentiation of resident leukocytes.

Abnormalities in molecules known to have important roles in decidualization, identified by chorionic villus sample (CVS) analysis from the first trimester, have been associated with the later development of pregnancy disorders linked to placental insufficiency. It is interesting to speculate whether abnormal decidualization in the peri-implantation period may be useful in identifying women at risk of implantation and pregnancy disorders.

2.4 The Uterine Fluid Microenvironment during the Peri-Implantation Period

2.4.1 Soluble Factors

Uterine fluid contains soluble factors and microvesicles that are important regulators of endometrial and blastocyst development and blastocyst–endometrial communication, all key for successful implantation. These soluble factors likely change throughout the menstrual cycle. In a non-conception cycle, factors present in uterine fluid are derived from a number of sources, including the endometrial glandular and luminal epithelium, selective transudation from blood, and likely from Fallopian tube secretions and peritoneal fluid. Moreover, in a conception cycle blastocyst secretions will also be present in uterine fluid in the peri-implantation phase. Uterine fluid also contains bacterial factors making up the microbiome, which is also thought to be important for implantation. The many different soluble factors present in uterine fluid include proteins, steroids, lipids, amino acids, simple salts, and noncoding RNA. Similarly, extracellular vesicles present in uterine fluid contain proteins, lipids, and nucleic acids including noncoding RNA. Many of these factors, including proteins and noncoding RNA, are secreted from the endometrium or blastocyst and facilitate endometrial–blastocyst communication and implantation [15].

Proteins present in uterine fluid include the cytokines LIF, VEGF, IL11, and other chemokines and proteases that are at least partly synthesized in the endometrium and secreted into the uterine cavity [15]. While a number of factors have been identified in uterine fluid, there have not been many studies that have determined their functional significance in embryo implantation.

2.4.2 Extracellular Vesicles

Extracellular vesicles, including exosomes (30–150 μm) and larger microvesicles (150–~300 μm), are released into the extracellular space by most cells and taken up by cells, thereby altering their function. While this has been extensively studied in cancer, recent studies are also examining the role of microvesicles, in particular exosomes, in implantation.

Exosomes are present in human uterine lavage and aspirate, and are at least partly released from the endometrial epithelium. Additionally, it is likely that microvesicles present in uterine fluid also originate from blood and other tissues in the female reproductive tract, and in a conception cycle, from blastocysts. There is clearly a complex interplay between the source and uptake of microparticles in the female reproductive tract, and recent studies are beginning to tease out these interactions. Endometrial exosome content varies across the menstrual cycle as steroid hormone-regulated proteins have been identified in endometrial exosomes. This implies that exosomes may be useful as biomarkers of endometrial maturation and receptivity.

Exosomes in uterine fluid are likely taken up by human blastocysts. A recent report revealed that exosomes were taken up by mouse trophectoderm. Furthermore, a specific miR, has-miR-30d, is present in exosomes in human uterine fluid; both exosome-associated and free has-miR-30d were internalized by mouse embryos, resulting in indirect over-expression of genes encoding for certain molecules associated with embryo adhesion. Functionally, exosomes secreted from the human endometrial epithelial cell carcinoma cell line ECC1, when taken up by the trophoblast cell line, HTR8, increased the adhesive capacity of the HTR8 cells, indicating that endometrial-derived exosomes may regulate human blastocyst implantation potential [16].

2.5 Embryo–Endometrial Interaction during Implantation

2.5.1 Key Molecules and Pathways Known to Participate in Embryo Apposition and Attachment

The initial embryo–endometrial interaction during human implantation remains largely unknown because it is impossible to study this process for obvious ethical reasons. Current understanding is thus drawn from in vitro models, histological examinations, and inference from other animal studies. The process is believed to begin with a weak and transient interaction between the blastocyst and the endometrial surface. It is proposed that the L-selectin adhesion system that blood leukocytes utilize to adhere to the vessel wall is shared by the human blastocyst to initiate the early interaction with the endometrium [17]. Once the blastocyst enters the uterine cavity, the free-floating sphere "rolls" on the endometrial surface and encounters the epithelial glycocalyx. The trophectoderm of hatched human blastocyst expresses L-selectin; this lectin-like protein recognizes specific sialylated or sulfated sugars such as sialyl Le-x and sialyl Le-y. Intriguingly, these specific carbohydrate structures are found to be carried by certain mucins such as mucin-1 on the apical surface of the endometrium. It is thus speculated that the interaction between L-selectin on the trophectoderm and L-selectin oligosaccharide ligands on the endometrial glycocalyx tethers the embryo and initiates the apposition stage of implantation [17].

This initial weak adhesion locates the embryo to a specific site and activates other molecules to establish firmer attachment. In vitro studies indicate that the attaching embryo secretes factors to induce local removal of mucin-1 beneath and adjacent to the embryo [10], which is then followed by firm adhesion of trophectoderm to non-mucin receptors on the endometrial epithelium. The ability of the attaching embryo to remove the mucin barrier has been speculated to function as a "health test" on the embryo [18].

Candidate adhesion systems that may mediate firm embryo attachment include the trophinin–tastin–bystin complex, heparin-binding EGF-like growth factor (HB-EGF) and its receptor ErbB4, and integrins [18]. Trophinin is a transmembrane glycoprotein that can elicit strong homophilic cell adhesion through trophinin–trophinin binding [19]. Human trophoblasts and endometrial epithelial cells that over-express trophinin adhere instantly in vitro [19]. Trophinin is expressed by both the trophectoderm and the apposed apical surface of luminal epithelium in rhesus monkey implantation sites [19]. There is evidence that human chorionic gonadotropin (hCG) secreted by the attaching human embryo induces trophinin expression in the endometrial epithelium for implantation [20]. Trophinin normally binds to its cytoplasmic partners bystin and tastin, and this complex further interacts with ErbB4 and suppresses its tyrosine kinase activity [21]. Trophinin–trophinin binding between adjacent cells is predicted to release bystin from the complex, and this dissociation acts as a switch to activate ErbB4 phosphorylation and the HB-EGF signaling pathway to trigger trophoblast invasion [21]. Integrins and their binding partners such as fibronectin, vitronectin, osteopontin, and possibly laminin have also been suggested to be important for firm embryo adhesion [18]. In particular, integrin $\alpha v\beta 3$ is believed to mediate human implantation and aberrant $\alpha v\beta 3$ integrin is associated with unexplained infertility.

2.5.2 Embryo Invasion into the Stroma and Mechanisms that Safeguard Quality Implantation

After firm attachment, the embryo invades between epithelial cells and moves into the underlying stroma. Remarkably, this process does not cause epithelial cell apoptosis, and how this is controlled is unknown. Trophoblasts from the trophectoderm then rapidly proliferate and differentiate along villous and extravillous pathways to initiate placental development [1]. In particular, the extravillous trophoblasts invade and infiltrate both the endometrial stroma and arteries to ensure adequate blood supply to the placenta.

As human trophoblast invasion resembles tumor invasion, the decidua plays a critical role in tolerating as well as limiting trophoblast invasion. This balance is critically important, because excessive invasion will cause placenta accreta or choriocarcinoma, whereas inadequate invasion will lead to placental insufficiency and a spectrum of pregnancy complications, including miscarriage, intrauterine growth restriction, and preeclampsia [13]. Decidualization alters stromal cell cytoskeletal organization, extracellular matrix composition and distribution, cytokine/chemokine secretion, and cell responsiveness to external stimuli [13]. For instance, decidualization is associated with distinctive nucleus rounding, profound accumulation of glycogen and lipid droplets in the cytoplasm, significant changes in cell adhesion complex proteins and gap junctions, and marked increase in pericellular collagen IV, laminin, fibronectin, heparin sulfate proteoglycan, vimentin, and desmin [13]. These changes would collectively pose a barrier to trophoblast invasion. On the other hand, decidualization renders the stromal environment more supportive to trophoblast expansion. Decidual cells secrete many cytokines, chemokines, and growth actors, including high levels of prolactin and IGFBP-1, which are markers of decidualization and shown to stimulate trophoblast growth and invasion [13]. In addition, the decidua contains a large number of resident leukocytes that provide a chemoattractant microenvironment to promote trophoblast invasion. In particular, uterine NK cells produce cytokines and angiogenic factors that play a central role in spiral arterial remodeling.

An emerging concept suggests that the decidua also functions as a sensor of embryo quality [22]. Human decidual cells are found to respond differently to high-quality versus low-quality human embryos in coculture systems. When conditioned media from preimplantation human embryos are cocultured with decidualizing human endometrial stromal cells, media from competent embryos have little impact on decidual secretion or gene expression. In contrast, media from developmentally impaired embryos elicit a strong response in decidual cells. These media selectively inhibit decidual secretion of pro-implantation modulators such as LIF, IL-1β, CCL11, and HB-EGF [23]. Genome-wide analysis revealed that 449 decidual genes are markedly deregulated by conditioned media from poor-quality embryos, and the most severely affected candidate is HSC70, which is profoundly down-regulated [22]. HSC70 is a constitutively expressed member of the heat shock protein 70 family of molecular chaperones and plays a critical role in regulating protein folding and multi-protein complex assembly. The severe down-regulation of HSC70 in decidual cells is postulated to cause ER stress and cell cycle arrest, and these responses are suggested to function as a stress test to the timely disposal of poor-quality embryos.

Furthermore, in vitro studies suggest that the decidual cells themselves are motile and their movement actively assists tissue remodeling and trophoblast invasion [13]. In cell culture models, decidual cells selectively migrate toward high-grade but not low-grade human embryos, and this guided migration is mediated by trophoblast-secreted factors, including platelet-derived growth factors AA (PDGF-AA), PDGF-BB, and HB-EGF.

It is thus clear that the maternal decidua actively participates in human implantation; it functions much more broadly and diversely than just passively "curbing" trophoblast invasion. The concept of the decidua acting as a choosy maternal gatekeeper to safeguard quality implantation is an attractive paradigm; however, it is still new and requires further investigation and validation.

2.5.3 Blastocyst Regulation of Implantation

Accumulating evidence demonstrates that human embryos may influence implantation via the release of factors, including hormones and non-coding RNA. Ex vivo evidence shows that human blastocysts secrete small non-coding RNA and microRNA that may be taken up by human endometrial epithelial cells to alter their adhesive capacity. One specific microRNA, miR-661, was found to be released by human IVF embryos that failed to implant when transferred. Blastocyst hormonal factors are also prominent regulators of implantation. hCG is secreted by blastocysts attached to endometrial epithelium. In vivo, hCG infusion into the uterine cavity of women and baboons alters the production of LIF, VEGF, IL11, and prokineticin 1, which are important for endometrial receptivity [24].

The embryonic metabolome is also a source of multiple factors that may influence implantation. Lactate secreted by human embryos has been proposed as a critical mediator of implantation. Lactate promotes tissue disaggregation, loosening adhesion of epithelial cells that could facilitate blastocyst invasion [25].

These data denote the complex mechanisms by which human embryos facilitate implantation. The data also suggest that measurement of blastocyst-derived factors, including microRNA, may be useful in the identification of blastocysts destined to implant and may also serve as useful targets to regulate their implantation.

References

1. James JL, Carter AM, Chamley LW. Human placentation from nidation to 5 weeks of gestation. Part I: what do we know about formative placental development following implantation? *Placenta* 2012; 33:327–334.

2. Salamonsen LA, Nie G, Hannan N, Dimitriadis E. Society for Reproductive Biology Founders' Lecture 2009. Preparing fertile soil: the importance of endometrial receptivity. *Reprod Fertil Dev* 2009; 21:923–934.

3. Evans J, Salamonsen LA, Winship A et al. Fertile ground: human endometrial programming and lessons in health and disease. *Nat Rev Endocrinol* 2016; 12:654–667.

4. Lindsay LA, Murphy CR. The cytoskeleton of uterine epithelial and stromal cells. In: Aplin JD, Fazleabas AT, Glasser SR, Giudice LC (eds.), *The Endometrium*, 2nd edn. London: Taylor and Francis; 2008: 66–75.

5. Murphy CR. The Cytoskeleton of uterine epithelial cells: a new player in uterine receptivity and the plasma membrane transformation. *Hum Reprod Update* 1995; 1:567–580.

6. Quinn CE, Casper RF. Pinopodes: a questionable role in endometrial receptivity. *Hum Reprod Update* 2009; 15:229–236.

7. Heng S, Cervero A, Simon C et al. Proprotein convertase 5/6 is critical for embryo implantation in women: regulating receptivity by cleaving EBP50, modulating ezrin binding, and membrane-cytoskeletal interactions. *Endocrinology* 2011; 152:5041–5052.

8. Carson DD, Bagchi I, Dey SK et al. Embryo implantation. *Dev Biol* 2000; 223:217–237.

9. Meseguer M, Pellicer A, Simón C. MUC1 and endometrial receptivity. *Mol Hum Reprod* 1998; 4:1089–1098.

10. Meseguer M, Aplin JD, Caballero-Campo P et al. Human endometrial mucin MUC1 is up-regulated by progesterone and down-regulated in vitro by the human blastocyst. *Biol Reprod* 2001; 64:590–601.

11. Heng S, Paule SG, Li Y et al. Posttranslational removal of α-dystroglycan N terminus by PC5/6 cleavage is important for uterine preparation for embryo implantation in women. *The FASEB Journal* 2015; 29:4011–4022.

12. Ruan YC, Chen H, Chan HC. Ion channels in the endometrium: regulation of endometrial receptivity and embryo implantation. *Hum Reprod Update* 2014; 20:517–529.

13. Gellersen B, Brosens JJ. Cyclic decidualization of the human endometrium in reproductive health and failure. *Endocrine Reviews* 2014; 35:851–905.

14. Dimitriadis E, White CA, Jones RL, Salamonsen LA. Cytokines, chemokines and growth factors in endometrium related to implantation. *Hum Reprod Update* 2005; 11:613–630.

15. Salamonsen LA, Evans J, Nguyen HPT, Edgell TA. The microenvironment of human implantation: determinant of reproductive success. *Am J Reprod Immunol* 2016; 75:218–225.

16. Greening DW, Nguyen HPT, Elgass K, Simpson RJ, Salamonsen LA. Human endometrial exosomes contain hormone-specific cargo modulating trophoblast adhesive capacity: insights into endometrial-embryo interactions. *Biol Reprod* 2016; 94:38, 31–15.

17. Genbacev OD, Prakobphol A, Foulk RA et al. Trophoblast L-selectin-mediated adhesion at the maternal-fetal interface. *Science* 2003; 299:405–408.

18. Aplin JD, Ruane PT. Embryo–epithelium interactions during implantation at a glance. *Journal of Cell Science* 2017; 130:15–22.

19. Fukuda MN, Sugihara K. An integrated view of L-selectin and trophinin function in human embryo implantation. *J Obstet Gynaecol Res* 2008; 34:129–136.

20. Sugihara K, Kabir-Salmani M, Byrne J et al. Induction of trophinin in human endometrial surface epithelia by CGβ and IL-1β. *FEBS Letters* 2008; 582:197–202.

21. Sugihara K, Sugiyama D, Byrne J et al. Trophoblast cell activation by trophinin ligation is implicated in human embryo implantation. *Proc Natl Acad Sci USA* 2007; 104:3799–3804.

22. Brosens JJ, Salker MS, Teklenburg G et al. Uterine selection of human embryos at implantation. *Sci Rep* 2014; 4:3894.

23. Teklenburg G, Salker M, Molokhia M et al. Natural selection of human embryos: decidualizing endometrial stromal cells serve as sensors of embryo quality upon implantation. *PLoS ONE* 2010; 5:e10258.

24. Evans J, Catalano RD, Brown P et al. Prokineticin 1 mediates fetal-maternal dialogue regulating endometrial leukemia inhibitory factor. *FASEB journal* 2009; 23:2165–2175.

25. Gardner DK. Lactate production by the mammalian blastocyst: manipulating the microenvironment for uterine implantation and invasion? *Bioessays* 2015; 37:364–371.

Chapter 3

Protein Biomarkers of Endometrial Receptivity

Tracey A. Edgell

3.1 Endometrial Receptivity

The endometrium is a mucosal tissue lining the uterine cavity. The endometrium cyclically regenerates from any remaining basalis layer following menses. A regenerative proliferative phase occurs pre-ovulation in response to estrogen, followed by a transition to a post-ovulation secretory phase regulated by estrogen and progesterone. Within this secretory phase the endometrium attains a receptive state approximately on days 6–10 post-ovulation, termed the 'window of implantation', which is timed to coincide with the arrival of a blastocyst into the uterine cavity. At this time, molecular changes in the glands and luminal epithelium result in changes to their secretions into the uterine cavity. Uterine fluid is a complex histotroph containing nutrients, enzymes, cytokines, anti-proteases and transport proteins, along with other biologically active factors [1]; it provides support to and can modify certain characteristics of the pre-implantation blastocyst. Additional changes also occur to mucins, integrins and other adhesion molecules [2] at the luminal epithelial surface and within the epithelial cells from which the secretions arise (e.g. changes in junctional complexes, Ca^{++} regulators, growth factors, cytokines, chemokines and prostanoids) [3–6].

In in vitro fertilisation (IVF) cycles, the correct timing of embryo transfer is critical for a successful outcome. A synchronicity of embryo and endometrium is essential; hence, a day 2 or day 5 embryo requires transfer to an endometrium on the second or the fifth day respectively following its initial exposure to progesterone. Embryos, either frozen or thawed, are typically transferred at cleavage stage (day 2 or 3) or blastocyst stage (day 5). Claims of a premature rise in progesterone prior to administration of the human chorionic gonadotrophin (hCG) trigger in IVF cycles have been associated with reduced pregnancy rates in stimulated cycles, presumably reflecting an advancement of endometrial maturation relative to the developmental stage of the embryo. However, these findings were not corroborated in a meta-analysis by Venetis et al. [7] which concluded that a premature rise in progesterone is not correlated with pregnancy outcome.

The impact of ovarian stimulation on endometrial receptivity was reviewed in detail by Fatemi and Popovic-Todorovic [8]. It is evident that the hormonal treatments used to induce multiple follicles disturb the endometrium with premature secretory changes in the early secretory phase, followed by a dys-synchronous glandular and stromal differentiation in the mid-luteal phase, resulting in both inadequate receptivity and/or changes in its timing. A retrospective study comparing morphological and immunohistochemical features on the day of oocyte retrieval in women in stimulation cycles found that those women who became pregnant following embryo transfer in the same cycle had endometrium showing significantly less alterations in histological endometrial maturation and leukocyte populations than that of the women who did not become pregnant [9].

3.2 Testing for Receptivity

The accurate dating of endometrial development by histology is difficult and remains subjective. Given that endometrial receptivity is essential to establishing a pregnancy, a receptivity test would assist the fertility specialist in three ways. Firstly, women who have a history of multiple implantation failures despite the transfer of good-quality embryos are potentially subject to endometrial receptivity failure as the cause of their infertility. The ability to identify a receptivity disorder would aid the decision to continue costly and emotionally exhausting IVF treatment, and for the clinician to tailor their treatment to address their endometrial issue. This testing would in all likelihood occur during the expected receptive phase of a woman's natural menstrual cycle prior to her next IVF cycle. Repeat testing in controlled trials may allow assessment as to which treatments are most effective in optimising the endometrium.

Secondly is the application to all women undergoing IVF treatment. As discussed earlier, hormonal stimulation may have significant impact on morphology in that cycle, potentially reducing the functionality of the endometrium. Meta-analysis indicates greater success transferring embryos in a subsequent natural cycle than fresh transfer in the stimulated cycle [10]. These observations highlight that the super-physiological hormonal stimulation protocols are detrimental to endometrial receptivity. Hence, a receptivity assay performed in a stimulation cycle would permit the clinician to assess the likelihood of success if proceeding with a transfer within that cycle and would inform whether he/she should go ahead or advise the patient to freeze all suitable embryos. Clearly, in this situation there are two major requirements of the assay: it must not reduce the likelihood of embryo implantation, i.e. not damage the endometrium, and the assay must be completed in an acceptable time frame between sampling and the planned transfer.

Finally, a receptivity test may be adopted into the standard work-up assessment of new patients, identifying receptivity issues prior to commencing treatment. A suitably reliable assay would guide the future treatment of these women, indicating from the outset if a natural cycle transfer is likely to be successful, or whether gentle estrogen/progesterone treatment of the endometrium may enhance the chance of success.

The direct value of a receptivity assay to improving success rates among the IVF community is clear from the examples outlined earlier. However, it must also be remembered that endometrial therapeutics is a neglected area of research. The development of receptivity biomarkers will drive understanding of both the endometrial role and its defects, ultimately leading to a demand for endometrial-focussed therapeutics.

3.3 Requirements of Biomarkers

A true marker of receptivity should be reliable in both natural and stimulated cycles. Thus, it is essential that biomarker validation presents a robust analysis in both natural and stimulated cycles. Many biomarker discovery studies to date have utilised samples from women without uterine pathologies, e.g. fibroids and polyps. While this approach suits the discovery phase, it must be remembered that many women presenting for IVF do have such conditions; thus, for a receptivity assay to be applicable in the wider clinical setting, validation studies must be performed across a typical IVF cohort and sufficiently weighted.

While validation with randomised control studies is the ideal, it has to be acknowledged that such trials are difficult to recruit; hence, initial validation would likely be retrospective. However, it should still cover the three major validation requirements of temporal, geographical and domain. To date no endometrial receptivity biomarkers have been validated to this level; indeed, validation often is no more than proof of protein presence within a handful of endometrial tissues using immunohistochemistry.

Consideration must be given to the form of a receptivity test, e.g. tissue, uterine fluid or serum, and the timing of sample collection. In patient assessment cycles there is a clear opportunity to sample tissue and to do so at any chosen time point of the cycle. However, during an IVF cycle tissue sampling potentially damages the endometrium and compromises successful embryo implantation. In these circumstances it is clear that sampling of uterine fluid from within the uterine cavity, or even serum, provides a more attractive, less invasive option. Final consideration is timing. Clearly following sampling, sufficient time is required to perform analysis, and consider results before proceeding to transfer or freeze embryos.

3.4 Biomarker Identification

In recent years, the simultaneous measurement of multiple markers to account for molecular complexity is becoming the standard in many fields, including cancers. With regard to endometrial receptivity, defects probably do represent a range of molecular changes, making it imperative that a large panel of biomarkers is available.

Over the past two decades the emergence of proteomic and multiplexing technologies has seen their application to endometrial receptivity studies. Studies have taken a variety of forms with variations in sample type (tissue, uterine fluid, serum) and cohort selection. The dynamic nature of the endometrium makes the sampling of material difficult with daily changes to the cellular and secretory composition. Comparisons have been made of the changes between proliferative and mid-secretory phases of fertile women [11–15], pre-receptive and receptive fertile women [16–18], or alternatively comparisons of mid-secretory samples (based on Noyes criteria) from fertile and infertile women with idiopathic infertility [13,19] or on the basis of outcome of embryo transfer in IVF [6]. Discovery has been driven by proteomic analysis, multiplex technologies or single identified protein studies, with immunohistochemistry, ELISA and functional assays being the staple validation methodologies. The advantage of proteomic and multiplex technologies has been the ability to differentially identify a vast number of molecular changes in matched samples; the disadvantage is that they have generated large lists of 'potential' markers, for which validation has been limited or non-existent. It should be noted that many of the published studies were performed early in the development of proteomics technologies, often using patient pools as opposed to individual samples and employing basic analysis by 2D gel and mass-spectrometry analysis. It may be expected that the results of these studies will not be upheld when extended to larger validation studies of individuals, and that a more advanced proteomic analysis of individual samples would potentially provide a more useful analysis.

3.4.1 Tissue Biomarkers

A number of studies have examined human endometrial tissue; tissue sampling is performed by pipelle biopsy or curettage. This is invasive [20] particularly for nulliparous women and may damage the endometrium. Endometrial receptivity or failure cannot be identified by tissue morphology alone, except when the endometrium is clearly inadequately developed for the expected phase of the menstrual cycle, e.g. insufficient thickness, lack of secretory features of glands and spiral arteriole development. A major limitation has been the abundant structural proteins inherent to tissue analysis; these proteins can mask low-abundance regulatory proteins.

Integrins are a class of cell adhesion molecules (CAMs), which include CD44, trophinin, $\alpha v \beta 3$ integrin and cadherin-11, which have also been investigated as playing a role in endometrial receptivity [21]. Among these, $\alpha v \beta 3$ integrin is the most promising, with its reduced expression of $\alpha v \beta 3$ linked with unexplained IVF failure, while upregulation has been associated with future IVF success. The CAM molecules interact with other CAMs, extracellular matrix proteins and matrix metalloproteinases. The expression of integrins is altered in many inflammatory conditions associated with implantation failure, e.g. endometriosis, hydrosalpinges and polycystic ovarian syndrome.

A number of proteomic studies of endometrial tissue have been published; the more significant proteins identified to date are listed in Table 3.1. In a two-dimensional, differential gel electrophoresis (2D-DiGE)-based study, Chen et al. [11] identified 196 differentially expressed protein spots between proliferative and secretory phases of fertile women. Perhaps not surprisingly, the majority of increased expressions were observed in the secretory phase endometrial samples. These spots often appeared in 'spot trains', the result of differing post-translational modifications (phosphorylation, glycosylation) of a single gene product, hence with differing molecular weight and pI values. A number of the proteins were proven by immunohistochemistry to be present in endometrial epithelial cells, and showed differing levels between proliferative and secretory tissues.

Table 3.1 Significant biomarkers discovered by proteomic studies of endometrial tissue. P = proliferative, MP = mid-proliferative, MS = mid-secretory

Biomarker	Study comparison	Reference
Chloride intracellular channel protein 1	MP vs. MS, fertile women	[11]
Rho GDP-dissociation inhibitor 1		
Membrane-associated progesterone receptor component 1		
Ezrin		
Glutamate NMDA receptor subunit zeta 1	P vs. MS	[12]
Proto-oncogene FRAT1		
Stathmin 1	Pre-receptive vs. receptive, fertile women	[16]
Annexin A2		
Annexin IV	Pre-receptive vs. receptive, fertile women	[17]

Dominguez et al. [16] also performed a 2D-DiGE study, this time of LH+2 versus LH+7 fertile women. The study identified a total of 32 differentially expressed proteins, of which just two (Annexin A2 and Stathmin I) were consistently regulated in dual experiments. The dual experimental design of this study highlights the inconsistencies associated with the 2D-DiGE analysis of a complex tissue. Analysis of entire endometrial biopsies for protein, or indeed genomic material, is confounded by the considerable variability in the proportions of epithelial cells to stromal fibroblasts, cells of the vasculature and leukocytes. The study of Chen et al. highlighted this issue as the protein coronin 1 was identified as upregulated in the proteomic analysis of secretory phase endometrium; however, validation by immunohistochemistry found it to be wholly contained in leukocyte populations and not the endometrial epithelial, stromal or vasculature [11]. Additionally, as demonstrated by histological assessment of stimulated (IVF) endometria, different cellular compartments (e.g. epithelium and stroma) may be 'out of phase' with each other, adding to the complication of such whole tissue analyses [9]. Laser capture of individual cell types provides a tool to overcome this complexity; however, its utility is limited by the very low yield of protein it provides, thus limiting proteomic identifications.

3.4.2 Uterine Fluid Biomarkers

Uterine fluid is a protein-rich histotroph comprising secretions from the endometrial glands, cleavage products of both the secreted proteins and glycocalyx (a glycoprotein mucin-rich layer coating the apical surface of the epithelium). This fluid provides the microenvironment for blastocyst development and implantation. The glandular secretions have been demonstrated in gland knockout animal models to be essential for implantation to occur. Thus, it is evident that analysis of uterine fluid should provide biomarkers of endometrial receptivity, and indeed faulty endometrial protein expression. However, uterine fluid does contain many abundant serum proteins (e.g. albumin) whose presence may be due to direct endometrial secretion, transudation from the blood vessels of the endometrium or contamination during the sample collection process. These proteins complicate analysis introducing an element of doubt as to their endometrial relevance. Furthermore, they may mask the less abundant proteins and have, in many studies, been a limiting factor on the depth of the proteome identified. Unfortunately, sample processing techniques to remove abundant proteins, (e.g. affinity removal using MARS columns) may give rise to an additional error in any quantitative analysis of identified proteins.

Collection of uterine fluid can take two forms, either aspiration or lavage collection; both are less invasive than tissue sampling. There is only a small volume of fluid (<10 μl retrieved by aspiration) present within the uterine cavity, and often aspirates will contain blood indicating damage to the tissue and compromising integrity of the sample. Uterine lavage is collected by gently infusing and retrieving 2–3 ml of saline into the uterine cavity so that it washes over the entire endometrial surface. Importantly, aspiration and lavage are not interchangeable for the purpose of analyte analysis [22], presumably because soluble analytes are released from the endometrial glycocalyx during lavage. Aspiration may be the better technique if sampling is to be performed in the same cycle as embryo transfer, as it does not appear to influence implantation rates [23]. However, as indicated earlier, collection of an aspirate does carry a risk of tissue damage within the uterus and may therefore compromise the endometrium at the time of implantation.

Proteomic approaches have provided a more detailed knowledge as to the contents of the uterine cavity than we previously appreciated. Casado-Vela [24] utilised three approaches in the analysis of uterine fluid, to reveal a total of 803 proteins, highlighting the complexity of the intra-uterine environment. Studies have identified differences between proliferative or early secretory phase and mid-secretory phase [14,19] and between mid-secretory phases of fertile and infertile women [19], summarised in Table 3.2. Notably, across these studies a number of broad activity anti-proteases were identified; notably, alpha-1-antitrypsin,

Table 3.2 Significant biomarkers discovered by proteomic studies of endometrial fluid. P = proliferative, MP = mid-proliferative, MS = mid-secretory. Bold type indicate proteins identified in multiple reports

Biomarker	Study comparison	Sample type	Reference
Apolipoprotein A1	P vs. MS, fertile women	Lavage	[14]
Apolipoprotein AIV			
Alpha-1-antitrypsin			
Alpha-1-antitrypsin	Pre-receptive (LH+4) vs. Receptive (LH+9), fertile women	Lavage	[18]
Kininogen 1			
78 kd glucose-regulated protein			
Glutathione transferase			
Apolipoprotein A1			
Transferrin			
Alpha-2-macroglobulin	MP vs. MS, fertile women	Lavage	[19]
Alpha-1-antitrypsin			
Interalpha-trypsin inhibitor family heavy chain-related protein			
Activin receptor type-2B			
Transthyretin	MS fertile vs. MS infertile women	Lavage	[19]
Antithrombin-III			
Vitamin D-binding protein			
Alpha-1-antichymotrypsin			
Alpha-1-antitrypsin			
Apolipoprotein A-I			
Apolipoprotein A-IV			
Activin receptor type-2B			
Alpha-2-macroglobulin			
PRSS3			
Angiotensinogen			

common to all three studies, was reduced in the mid-secretory phase. Anti-thrombin III and alpha-2-macroglobulin were the only proteins validated by examination of their presence in endometrial tissue. Both were found to be epithelial products indicative of their source being secretion from the endometrium. Looking to the future it is noted that many of the identified proteins appeared as spot trains in the 2D-gel analysis, and, as such, we may expect that future more detailed analysis of such forms may spread further light on their role and significance to receptivity and embryo implantation.

Multiplexing studies have investigated a variety of cytokine, chemokine and growth factors present in the uterine fluid [6,13]. These factors, commonly unseen in proteomic analysis, are key in determining cell behaviours. Multiplexing permits the detailed analysis of very small volumes of aspirate or lavage samples. In a study of aspirates collected prior to embryo transfer in women undergoing IVF, Boomsma reported from among a panel of 17 factors significant associations of monocyte chemoattractant protein-1 (MCP-1) interferon-gamma inducible 10kDa protein (IP-10) with implantation and interleukin 1-beta (IL-1beta) and tumour necrosis factor-alpha (TNF-alpha) with clinical pregnancy. Hannan and colleagues screened a panel of 42 cytokines and growth factors in lavage samples, collected during the proliferative and mid-secretory phases of fertile women, and compared these to the mid-secretory phase of idiopathic infertile women, in natural cycles. Though some 30 factors were detectable, no significant differences were seen between patient groups, likely a reflection of just $n=4$/group in the cohort.

3.4.3 Blood, Urine and Saliva

Clearly, a minimally invasive test based on blood, urine or saliva would be optimal, as testing need not be limited to days when the patient is in the clinic, and, indeed, consecutive days of testing to identify the optimal transfer time becomes possible. However, this presents a challenge since most of the factors identified as potential biomarkers are produced locally by the endometrium in very low concentrations and secreted into the uterine lumen, and it is questionable whether any would reach blood or urine.

One study that has examined serum was that of Bastu and colleagues in 2015 [25]. The authors examined serum collected during the implantation window (7–9 days post-LH surge) from women with a history of recurrent implantation failure for two biomarkers, Muc1 and glycodelin (formerly known as placental protein 14, PP14). Both proteins have previously been linked with sperm-zona interaction, endometrial receptivity and maintenance of pregnancy. The small study found lower concentration of both biomarkers in the serum of the implantation failure women compared to fertile controls.

More recently, as yet unpublished data have been presented by the Salamonsen laboratory. This combines a panel of six cytokine/chemokines into a multivariate algorithm for the prediction of fresh embryo transfer outcome in stimulated cycles. In a study of 280 women from whom blood was collected during oocyte retrieval, encouraging results of 100 per cent and 80 per cent correct prediction of implantation were obtained for day 3 and day 5 transfers respectively, within the stimulation cycle.

3.5 The Future

To achieve marked improvements in IVF outcomes, it is essential that predictive tests for endometrial receptivity are introduced into clinical practice. To date, no single biomarker has emerged for endometrial receptivity, and it seems likely that any future test will require multiple biomarkers; these may be drawn from the previously published analyses or future higher-powered proteomic studies, in conjunction with a minimally invasive and convenient sampling procedure. At this time, the potential emergence of an assay with sufficient performance in retrospective analyses may pave the way for a randomised control study, essential for any assay to reach clinical acceptability and commercial viability. We are rapidly approaching this possibility. Undoubtedly, future proteomic analyses, notably those that address post-translational modifications, may present the greatest progress.

Post-translational modifications, notably glycosylation and phosphorylation, have the potential to dramatically alter activity and efficiency of an individual protein. The early proteomic studies discussed earlier have highlighted the abundance and relevance of such variable modifications, evidenced as spot trains in 2D-DIGE studies. As we understand more of their role, we will see the need to exploit them as diagnostic indicators, driving pathology-appropriate assay design.

References

1. Leese, H.J. et al., Female reproductive tract fluids: composition, mechanism of formation and potential role in the developmental origins of health and disease. *Reprod Fertil Dev* 2008; **20**:1–8.

2. Quenby, S. et al., Different types of recurrent miscarriage are associated with varying patterns of adhesion molecule expression in endometrium. *Reprod Biomed Online* 2007; **14**:224–34.

3. Buck, V.U., et al., Redistribution of adhering junctions in human endometrial epithelial cells during the implantation window of the menstrual cycle. *Histochem Cell Biol* 2012; **137**:777–90.

4. Hannan, N.J., J. Evans, and L.A. Salamonsen, Alternate roles for immune regulators: establishing endometrial receptivity for implantation. *Expert Review of Clinical Immunology* 2011; **7**:789–802.

5. Luu, K.C., G.Y. Nie, and L.A. Salamonsen, Endometrial calbindins are critical for embryo implantation: evidence from in vivo use of morpholino antisense oligonucleotides. *Proc Natl Acad Sci USA* 2004; **101**:8028–33.

6. Boomsma, C.M. et al., Endometrial secretion analysis identifies a cytokine profile predictive of pregnancy in IVF. *Hum Reprod* 2009; **24**:1427–35.

7. Venetis, C. et al., Progesterone elevation and probability of pregnancy after IVF: a systematic review and meta-analysis of over 60,000 cycles. *Human Reprod Update* 2013; **19**:433–457.

8. Fatemi, H.M. and B. Popovic-Todorovic, Implantation in assisted reproduction: a look at endometrial receptivity. *Reprod Biomed Online* 2013; **27**:530–8.

9. Evans, J. et al., Defective soil for a fertile seed? Altered endometrial development is detrimental to pregnancy success. *PLoS One* 2012; **7**:e53098.

10. Roque, M. et al., Fresh embryo transfer versus frozen embryo transfer in in vitro fertilization cycles: a systematic review and meta-analysis. *Fertil Steril* 2013; **99**:156–62.

11. Chen, J.I. et al., Proteomic characterization of midproliferative and midsecretory human endometrium. *Journal of Proteome Research* 2009; **8**:2032–44.

12. DeSouza, L. et al., Proteomic analysis of the proliferative and secretory phases of the human endometrium: protein identification and differential protein expression. *Proteomics* 2005; **5**:270–81.

13. Hannan, N.J. et al., Analysis of fertility-related soluble mediators in human uterine fluid identifies VEGF as a key regulator of embryo implantation. *Endocrinology* 2011; **152**:4948–56.

14. Parmar, T. et al., Protein repertoire of human uterine fluid during the mid-secretory phase of the menstrual cycle. *Hum Reprod* 2008; **23**:379–86.

15. Salamonsen, L.A. et al., Proteomics of the human endometrium and uterine fluid: a pathway to biomarker discovery. *Fertil Steril* 2013; **99**:1086–92

16. Dominguez, F. et al., Proteomic analysis of the human receptive versus non-receptive endometrium using differential in-gel electrophoresis and MALDI-MS unveils stathmin 1 and annexin A2 as differentially regulated. *Human Reproduction* 2009; **24**: 2607–17.

17. Li, J. et al., [Study of altered expression of annexin IV and human endometrial receptivity]. *Zhonghua Fu Chan Ke Za Zhi* 2006; **41**:803–5.

18. Scotchie, J.G. et al., Proteomic analysis of the luteal endometrial secretome. *Reproductive Sciences* 2009; **16**:883–93.

19. Hannan, N.J. et al., 2D-DiGE analysis of the human endometrial secretome reveals differences between receptive and nonreceptive states in fertile and infertile women. *Journal of Proteome Research* 2010; **9**:6256–64.

20. Nastri, C. et al., Endometrial injury in women undergoing assisted reproductive techniques. *Cochrane Database Syst Rev* 2015; Mar 22; **3**:CD009517. doi: 10.1002/ 14651858.CD009517.pub3.

21. Lessey, B.A., Endometrial integrins and the establishment of uterine receptivity. *Hum Reprod* 1998; **13**:247–58.

22. Hannan, N.J. et al., Uterine lavage or aspirate: which view of the intrauterine environment? *Reproductive Sciences* 2012; **19**:1125–32.

23. van der Gaast, M.H. et al., Endometrial secretion aspiration prior to embryo transfer does not reduce implantation rates. *Reprod Biomed Online* 2003; **7**: 105–9.

24. Casado-Vela, J. et al., Comprehensive proteomic analysis of human endometrial fluid aspirate. *Journal of Proteome Research* 2009; **8**:4622–32.

25. Bastu, E. et al., Role of Mucin 1 and Glycodelin A in recurrent implantation failure. *Fertil Steril* 2015; **103**:1059–64.

Genetic Markers of Endometrial Receptivity

Patricia Díaz-Gimeno and Juan A. Garcia-Velasco

4.1 Endometrial Receptivity and Biomarkers: A Brief Introduction

In assisted reproductive techniques (ARTs), the endometrium is a main factor for embryo implantation. Therefore, it is very important to evaluate endometrial receptivity in the reproductive medicine context.

The endometrium is a highly dynamic tissue with a molecular timing related to the progression of the menstrual cycle. The menstrual cycle period when the embryo is able to implant is called the window of implantation (WOI) and the endometrial phenotype is called endometrial receptivity [1]. Endometrial receptivity acquisition is characterized for cellular and molecular changes in the mid-secretory phase, which configures such a complex and multifactorial process. All these changes are regulated mainly by ovarian steroid hormones, cytokines, chemokines, and other paracrine molecules, and lot of functions related to cell cycle division, immune system, or growth factors are implicated.

The first menstruation day is the reference point and day 0 of the cycle. During the proliferative phase, the endometrial oestrogen levels increase progressively, causing the proliferation of stromal and glandular cells, the elongation of spiral arteries, the development of cilia on epithelial cells, and mitotic activity in fibroblasts. In addition, progesterone is released by the corpus luteum after ovulation, causing several morphological changes in the endometrium, which acquires a receptive phenotype during the mid-secretory phase. When implantation does not occur, the progesterone and oestrogen levels decrease and the secretory stage finishes, restarting a new cycle (Figure 4.1).

All the levels of analysis explored and parameters studied have distinguished between a proliferative and secretory endometrium. The difficulty has been in distinguishing exactly the mid-secretory phase and a functional endometrial receptivity status from the subfertility one. At the tissue level, histology has been the gold standard for endometrial dating since the 1950s, providing a subjective diagnostic technique for the mid-secretory phase definition. This standard is based in Noyes criteria, which has defined a multifactorial histological approach considering eight histological parameters: gland mitosis, pseudo-stratification of nuclei, basal vacuolation, secretion, stromal oedema, pseudo-decidual reaction, stromal mitoses, and leukocyte infiltration. The accuracy and reproducibility of the histological criteria for mid-secretory phase have been largely questioned in clinical trials. These discussions conclude that Noyes criteria do not provide objective and useful clinical information to guide embryo transfer and are not related to fertility status.

From a cellular perspective, scanning electron microscopy with high resolution distinguishes the plasma membrane transformation with the emergence of pinopodes and

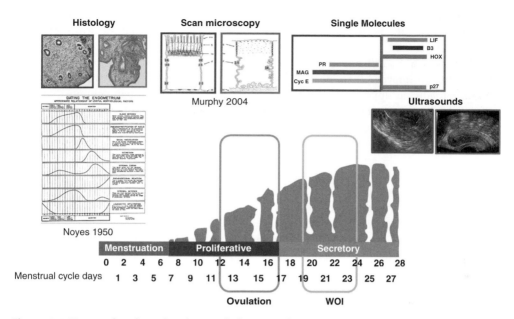

Figure 4.1 Menstrual cycle and endometrial changes. After menstruation, the proliferative endometrium increases in thickness and the secretory phase follows ovulation. Ovulation days vary by population depending on the LH behaviour and the endometrial receptivity status is opened in a period of time called WOI during the secretory phase. The different biomarkers distinguish accurately between a proliferative and a secretory endometrium (left side and right side of each approach, respectively) but not the endometrial receptivity optimal profile. From the left- to the right-upper part of the image: histology slides guided by Noyes, cellular morphology, single molecules proposed for each phase, and the ultrasounds non-trilaminar and trilaminar endometrium

adhesion molecule changes. Despite pinopodes appearing as cellular surface structures in the secretory phase, they are not sufficiently consistent as biomarkers of endometrial receptivity, and scanning microscopy is not a useful technology for daily diagnosis. Clinical advances in the field incorporate ultrasonographic features of the endometrium as uterine contractility, but the search for biomarkers at this level remains contradictory. The search for single molecular approaches which can predict endometrial receptivity, like HOXA10, MUC1, beta-3 integrin, or the regulation of cyclin E and p27, has failed since the 1990s. This fact is not surprising considering that implantation is a complex and multi-factorial process, and the classic Noyes criteria highlight endometrial dating as a multiparametric process.

In the twentieth century, medicine experienced a transition from anatomical to molecular medicine, and now in the twenty-first century from molecular to genomic medicine. In the last 20 years, new technologies have been developed that allow researchers to characterize complex fertility traits.

4.2 Genomics and Precision Medicine

Medicine is experiencing big changes fostered by new technologies that open to us different levels for understanding in clinical research and practice. During the last 20 years, genomics has become a key for characterizing multifactorial complex traits. Since the development of microarray technology in 1996 and the human genome draft publication in 2003, we can characterize molecular processes from the genomic point of view. This means that we are able to gather all the information about the whole transcriptome and the sequence of the entire genome. The use of this knowledge in the field of medicine is called genomic medicine, which is a different approach to genetic medicine, which uses knowledge about single genes to improve the diagnosis and treatment of single-gene disorders. The term 'genomic medicine' appeared in 2003 after the first draft of the human genome. Now our increased understanding of the interactions between the entire genome and non-genomic factors that result in health and disease is paving the way for an era of 'genomic medicine', in which new diagnostic and therapeutic approaches to common multifactorial conditions are emerging [2].

Genomic medicine provides a better definition of molecular diseases and a deeper understanding of diseases based on these massive data generated by genomic technologies. These findings inevitably necessitate reclassification of disease states, resulting in the development of a 'New Taxonomy of Disease' and generating a medicine with more precision [3]. The terms 'personalized medicine', 'stratified medicine', and 'precision medicine' are the consequence of applying this genomic knowledge where patients are subclassified or stratified, enabling more accurate clinical protocols for each subtype. Currently, the WHO recognizes the role of human genomics research and related biotechnologies in health (www.who.int/genomics/about/en/), and genomics is providing a source for patient stratification and for sub-phenotyping diseases.

The evolution of statistics and bioinformatic approaches applied to genomic data and its interpretation have been key for genomic medicine research advances, translation, and clinical application. Of considerable importance has been the analysis of genomic complexity from a systems biology point of view and by using specialized approaches for massive data analysis.

Systems biology views biology as an information science, which studies biological systems and its interactions with the environment or context. The systems genomics approach has considerable power in the search for informative diagnostic biomarkers of diseases because it focuses on the fundamental causes and keys for identification and understanding of disease-perturbed molecular networks. The importance of understanding network structure and dynamics is a main point in comparison to the single approach of molecular biology [4]. Network models are based on mathematical graph theory and provide an information base approach to model molecular information. Network medicine is a new discipline applied to human diseases with the potential to generate hypotheses and to predict biomarkers and functions [5].

Currently, thanks to the big genomic projects, we have available genomic sample databases as GEO (www.ncbi.nlm.nih.gov/gds/) or SRA (www.ncbi.nlm.nih.gov/sra/) for transcriptomics data, or IGSR (www.internationalgenome.org/), ExAC (http://exac.broadinstitute.org/), and TGCA (https://cancergenome.nih.gov/) for genome-sequencing data. Other databases of genomic knowledge are related to biological functions and disease processes as gene ontology (GO), Kyoto Encyclopaedia of Genes and Genomes (KEGG), or Reactome. We can also find powerful drug response databases to map the target pathways to a wide number of generic drug groups and their associated molecules and reported side effects [6]. One of the drug targets databases is included in KEGG as KEGG Drug section, or DrugBank. All this information can be interconnected and provides an opportunity to generate molecular models based on representative and powerful scientific knowledge and a source of new hypotheses.

Systems medicine is a systems approach focused on a holistic understanding of complex biomedical systems. It is based on the application of information technology to increasingly understand sets of clinical, molecular, cellular, phenotypic, demographic, and psycho-cognitive patient data. This approach is also called P4 medicine, because it creates effective predictive, personalized, preventive, and participatory models to treat patients. Nowadays, P4 medicine has been transformed into P5 medicine, including as a fifth P the 'psycho-cognitive' aspects to be considered to empower the patient, increase his/her quality of life, and transform him/her from a passive recipient into an active decision-maker. The fifth P analyses the behavioural component based on the way individuals act to prevent, cope, and react to illnesses and how they decide between different therapeutic options and interact with clinicians in the treatment process [7]. All this patient information from a P5 medicine approach is a new way to perform medical practices and to develop smart health strategies, and will transform the healthcare sector and society by providing safe and cost-effective treatments. Systems biology is a key aspect of P5 medicine, providing the methodological context to achieve P5 medicine objectives.

Computer technologies are a key element in systems medicine that provide tools and strategies for managing and analysing heterogeneity and large biological and patient environmental data sets (molecular 'omics', imaging, clinical, demographic, psycho-cognitive, etc.).

4.3 Genomic Approaches in Medicine

One of the most useful approaches in genomic medicine includes transcriptomic predictors, functional analysis, network modelling, and drug response models.

Transcriptomic predictors have been applied to genomic medicine as powerful tools for stratifying patients and sub-phenotype diseases, for improving diagnosis, and in the personalization of treatments. Since the advent of the first predictors [8], the guidelines and best practices have been defined, updated, and approved by the Food and Drug Administration for medical diagnosis [9]. These steps ensure that transcriptomic predictors will continue to make valuable contributions to clinical treatment.

Such predictors are generated computationally by machine learning from microarray data for known samples, to make predictions for unknown samples. Machine learning uses a data matrix, called a training set, as a reference. Predictors classify unknown samples learning from the training set. The training set is a model sample set that should be carefully defined and phenotyped because it is critical for the predictor's design.

The theoretical rule underlying predictors is that if the differences between classes are a consequence of certain differences at a transcriptomic level, then it is possible to find patterns of differences and use them to classify a new sample related to its gene expression. Finding ways to detect these differences is not always as simple as a linear solution, and there are sophisticated mathematical strategies that are designed for this purpose.

The most important aspect in the learning process is the self-assessment of prediction performance (Figure 4.2A). The self-assessment process is where error estimation for the model is calculated and all the prediction performance parameters defined as sensitivity and specificity. This statistical procedure consists in dividing the training data randomly into blinded and non-blinded portions and using the blinded prediction to estimate the error. Each part of the data must contain a fair representation of the classes to be learned. Then,

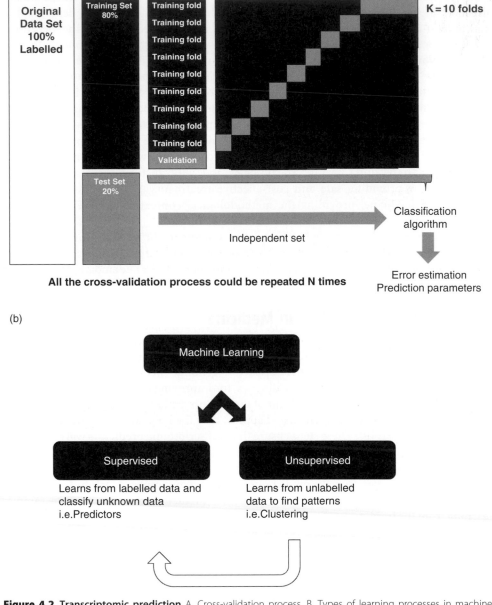

Figure 4.2 Transcriptomic prediction A. Cross-validation process. B. Types of learning processes in machine learning. Unsupervised learning could be used as supervision criteria for predictors learning

one of the parts (fold) is blinded (the test set) and the rest of the folds (the training set) are used to train the classifier. Then, the efficiency of the classifier is calculated using the corresponding test set which has not been used for the training of the classifier in this cross-validation. This complete process is repeated as many times as the number of partitions performed and, finally, an average of the efficiency of classification is obtained.

The learning process can occur from a labelled training set (supervised learning, i.e., transcriptomic predictors) or by using an unlabelled microarray set to structure data and define profiles (unsupervised learning, i.e., clustering methods). Sometimes unsupervised learning can be used to supervise the training set for transcriptomic predictors, as was done for a breast cancer risk prognostic signature providing a new taxonomy for diseases. Predictor design, especially the training set population inference and how it is supervised, is key for good model performance (Figure 4.2B).

In the reproductive field, some preliminary transcriptomic models have been implemented in embryo aneuploidy and in granulosa cells as predictive for embryo quality. However, the most extensive application of transcriptomic predictors in reproduction has been for other complex and multifactorial contributors to infertility, such as the endometrial factor.

4.4 Functional Analysis, Network Modelling, and Drug Response Models

Transcriptomics describes gene activity; therefore, concurrent functional analysis is key for understanding the underlying biology. Early functional analysis involved mapping expressed genes onto pathways such as KEGG pathways or functional ontologies such as GO. Nowadays, functional analysis has developed a new perspective, based on systems biology, which considers the functional interdependency of the molecular components of human cells; therefore, a disease is rarely a consequence of a single gene abnormality. Functional analysis involves genes in the genomic and cellular context and has recently expanded into three main approaches: functional enrichment analysis that highlights and ranks biologically relevant pathways, processes, disease markers, or other functionality in a gene list, biological network reconstruction, and interactome analysis [10].

Gene set enrichment analysis (GSEA) analyses functions by considering genes either in a genomic or cellular context. The genes are ranked by any biological criteria (e.g. differential expression between experimental cohorts and healthy controls) and the algorithm searches for blocks of functionally related genes without imposing any artificial thresholds as FC or adjusted p value.

Network science models 'simplify' systems biology complex systems into components (nodes: molecules) and interactions (edges) based on different biological parameters and apply graph theory to generate systems properties (centrality, betweenness, degree, etc.) and to predict new hypotheses and proposed new biomarkers in the framework of network medicine principles. Depending on the relationship between these nodes, different types of networks could be defined, e.g. metabolic, protein–protein interaction, gene regulatory, gene co-expression, or interactome networks [10].

In gene co-expression networks, also called co-expression networks, nodes represent genes and edges link pairs of genes that show co-expression above a set threshold. Common signalling cascades of gene products or protein complexes that function together are expected to show more similarities in their expression behaviour than random sets of gene products.

Drug network models are a representative system based on drug target effects from a systems biology perspective. Drug response models using genomics have been applied in other fields of medicine such as cardiovascular drugs [6]. This application is very powerful to new drug designs and to predict possible side effects. In the field of reproductive medicine, this approach is a model still unexplored.

4.5 Endometrial Factor Evaluation in ARTs

Wilcox and colleagues timed the WOI as occurring between eight and ten days after ovulation, defined by measuring human chorionic gonadotrophin (hCG) in urine in conception cycles [1]. In natural cycles, the LH peak in blood has been used as the reference, considering the WOI is opened between LH+5 and LH+9, the gold standard considered

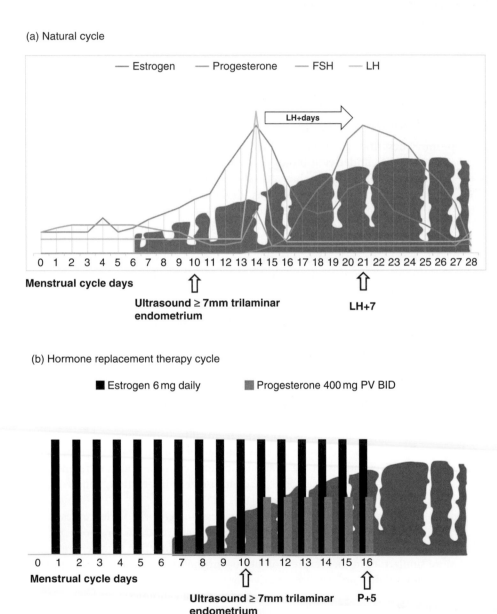

(a) Natural cycle

— Estrogen   — Progesterone   — FSH   — LH

LH+days

0 1 2 3 4 5 6 7 8 9 10 11 12 13 14 15 16 17 18 19 20 21 22 23 24 25 26 27 28

Menstrual cycle days

Ultrasound ≥ 7mm trilaminar endometrium

LH+7

(b) Hormone replacement therapy cycle

■ Estrogen 6 mg daily   ■ Progesterone 400 mg PV BID

0 1 2 3 4 5 6 7 8 9 10 11 12 13 14 15 16

Menstrual cycle days

Ultrasound ≥ 7mm trilaminar endometrium

P+5

Figure 4.3 Standard protocol for embryo transfer in natural cycle and in A. hormone replacement therapy; B. LH: luteinizing hormone; FSH: follicle-stimulation hormone

being LH+7. It has always been assumed that seven complete days after LH peak are necessary to reach the WOI, which then remains open for approximately two days (Figure 4.3A). Hormone replacement therapies (HRTs) comprise the administration of exogenous oestrogens and progesterone to control endometrial preparation for implantation. It has always been assumed that five complete days of progesterone administration in an HRT are necessary to reach the WOI (Figure 4.3B).

In both types of cycles, a trilaminar endometrium with a thickness of more than 7 mm before ovulation is often considered to predict a prepared endometrium for performing the embryo transfer in the expected WOI day (LH+7 or P+5).

However, considerable individual and menstrual inter-cycle variation has been reported in natural cycles and in HRT, and the standards are not working in part of the population.

4.6 Genomic Markers of Endometrium

As we can understand after this introduction, discussion about genetic markers of endometrial receptivity is essentially about genomics of endometrial receptivity and specifically about endometrial transcriptomics.

A transcriptomics approach, in comparison with other 'omic' approaches, provides the advantage to detect that environmental and genomic mutations are evidenced indirectly at the transcriptomic level. In addition, transcriptomics provision of biomarkers is the most reproducible and mature in terms of bioinformatics analysis. Guidelines for transcriptomic analysis are well established and the use of transcriptomic signatures as biomarkers has been approved and standardized by the FDA [9].

During the last 15 years, the gene expression profile of human endometrial receptivity has been widely investigated in natural cycles, controlled ovarian stimulation cycles, and refractory endometrium in patients with IUD by using microarrays technologies [11].

Table 4.1A Endometrial factor transcriptomic signature researches
The two types of endometrial factor transcriptomic signatures published. FC: fold change; d: menstrual cycle day; ES: early secretory endometrium; P: proliferative endometrium; LH+: days after luteinizing hormone peak

Type	Study	Day of biopsy	Threshold	Nº of genes
Receptivity	Kao et al.	d8–10 vs. LH+8–10	FC<2	533
Receptivity	Carson et al.	LH+2–4 vs. LH+7–9	FC<2	693
Receptivity	Riesewijk et al.	LH+2 vs. LH+7	FC<3	211
Receptivity	Borthwick et al.	d9–11 vs. LH+6–8	FC<2	136
Receptivity	Ponnampalam et al.	Complete cycle	FC<2	571
Receptivity	Mirkin et al.	LH+3 vs. LH+8	FC<2	107
Receptivity	Punyadeera et al.	d2–5 vs. d11–14	FC and p-value	54
Receptivity	Talbi et al.	P vs. ES	FC<2	648

Table 4.1A (cont.)

Type	Study	Day of biopsy	Threshold	N° of genes
RIF	Tapia et al.	Induced receptivity	FC<2	30
RIF	Bersinger et al.	d23.6 ± 1.8	FC<2	109
Receptivity	Haouzi et al.	LH+2 vs. LH+7	FC<2	1020
RIF	Koler et al.	d21	FC>2 and p value<0.05	313
RIF	Almäe et al.	LH+7	FC>3 and PFP<0.05	260
Receptivity	Diaz-Gimeno et al.	LH+1–5 vs. LH+7	Adj-p value<0.05/ FC>3	238
RIF	Bhagwat et al.	Complete cycle	Metanalysis score	179
RIF	Koot et al.	LH+5–8	Predictive value	303
RIF	Shi et al.	d5–7	Adj-p value<0.05	357

Table 4.1B Endometrial receptivity signature as gold standard in the research of endometrial effects in treatments or in pathological conditions. ERA: Endometrial Receptivity Analysis; RIF: recurrent implantation failure; MP: middle proliferative endometrium; ES: early secretory endometrium; MS: middle secretory endometrium; LS: late secretory endometrium. COS: controlled ovarian stimulation; COCP: combined oral contraceptive pill; hCG: human chorionic gonadotrophin; HRT: hormone replacement therapy; WOI: window of implantation

Author	Main outcome measured	Comparison
Diaz-Gimeno et al.	Dating by Noyes vs. ERA	MP vs. ES vs. MS vs. LS
Ruiz-Alonso et al.	RIF vs. Controls	pWOI/pWOIdelayed/pWOIadvanced
Bermejo et al.	COCP in COS	COS control vs. COS COCP
Nejat et al.	Diagnostic concordance	ERA vs. nuclear channel system
García-Velasco et al.	ERA endometriosis	Endometriosis vs. controls
Strug et al.	hCG effect in endometrial preparation	hCG vs. controls
Comstock et al.	HRT P+5	Obesity vs. controls
Diaz-Gimeno et al.	Expected WOI transcriptome	WOI sub-signatures clinical follow up

We can define as transcriptomic signature the genes and their related expression values that can together define a disease or process as a profile. Endometrial transcriptomic signatures can be divided into two main types.

Those studies designed to highlight signatures that can distinguish between a receptive versus non-receptive endometrium are called endometrial dating signatures or endometrial receptivity signatures; other signatures can distinguish between control versus pathological conditions, such as recurrent implantation failure (RIF), and pathological or disrupted signatures.

In Table 4.1A, endometrial factor signatures and the study design for the different two types of approaches are outlined.

4.7 Transcriptomic Predictors in Endometrial Factor

The first transcriptomic predictor in endometrial receptivity was built using the menstrual cycle days and the luteinizing hormone (LH) peak as a reference to supervising the training set.

The gene signature was selected following comparison between receptive (LH+7) and pre-receptive (LH+1–5) endometrial gene expression samples. After intersecting differential expressed genes (FDR<0.05, FC>3) from three independent methods, the most robust 238 genes were selected to build a customized array representative of receptivity [12]. This design focused on characterizing endometrial transcriptomics within the secretory phase.

After the gene selection, an independent cohort of samples across the menstrual cycle was used to train a transcriptomic predictor model and to define the menstrual cycle phases using this transcriptomic signature (endometrial dating model). On the other hand, the same signature was trained to detect an RIF profile (pathological model).

The endometrial dating model was trained using samples across the menstrual cycle from a healthy fertility-tested population, and the pathological model was trained with control versus RIF samples on the same LH day (LH+7). Endometrial Receptivity Analysis (ERA$_®$) focuses on recognizing the endometrial receptivity transcriptome; therefore, it is a balanced training set to distinguish between receptive and non-receptive status. In more detail, the training set was composed of 79 endometrial samples, proliferative (PF), pre-receptive (PR), and post-receptive (PS), with defined non-receptive ($n=40$) and receptive classes (R) ($n=39$) (Figure 4.4A). For the cycle dating in fertile women, each donor's endometrial sample was timed based on the LH peak determined from the menstrual cycle. This R ($n=39$) group was formed from samples obtained at day LH+7 and the PR ($n=14$) group from day LH+1 to LH+4. The PF group ($n=14$) included samples collected on day 8–12 of the menstrual cycle, and the post-secretory group ($n=12$) consisted of samples from LH+11 to LH+13. Cross-validation 10 folds and 5x stratified was implemented, dividing the cross-validation set into five balanced groups, leaving 1 out of 10 times as a test set. A specificity of 88.57 per cent and a sensitivity of 99.76 per cent for receptivity profile were obtained [12]. The pathological model was trained with control receptive samples (R) ($n=39$) and RIF patients ($n=11$), all of them collected in LH+7. The signature had no clear predictive value for distinguishing between RIF and controls (specificity of 0.65 and a sensitivity of 0.98) due to the heterogeneity in two main groups of RIF patients. Four of the RIF samples were reclassified as receptive and seven as RIF, and all the receptive samples were further classified. When we compared the RIF samples with the non-receptive control samples, some of them clustered with the pre-receptive ones showing

(a)

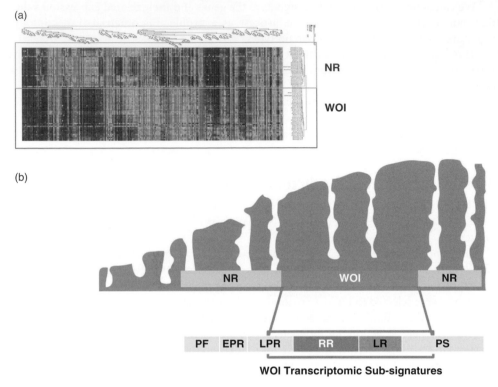

NR

WOI

(b)

NR   WOI   NR

PF   EPR   LPR   RR   LR   PS

WOI Transcriptomic Sub-signatures

Figure 4.4 **Endometrial receptivity signature** A. Supervised clustering by LH with the 238 most significant genes as predictive signature of endometrial receptivity; B. WOI transcriptomic stratification defines four transcriptomic sub-signatures associated with live birth and biochemical pregnancy. RR is the optimal receptivity and LR the transcriptomic profile associated with high-risk biochemical pregnancies

a displacement. The conclusion was that RIF samples were a heterogeneous group with both displaced and non-displaced samples [19, 14].

ERA test results were compared with Noyes histological criteria using the LH peak as gold standard to determine menstrual phases in a subset of samples (n=49). ERA classification by two independent pathologists was measured with concordance Kappa index [13]. Comparison between the histological dating performed by the two pathologists against the LH peak yielded Kappa index values of 0.681 (0.446–0.791) and 0.685 (0.545–0.824), respectively, and inter-observer variability (concordance between both pathologists) was 0.622 (0.435–0.839). The ERA test obtained a Kappa index of 0.922 (0.815–1.000), demonstrating that the ERA method is more objective and accurate than classic histology to date secretory phase.

Due to the results mentioned above, endometrial RIF was understood to be a transcriptomic displacement of the WOI. Different women may have differing transcriptomic profiles even if samples are taken on the same day or following the same hormonal treatment regimen [14]. The commercial and clinical application based on this procedure, for the personalization of embryo transfer day based on the transcriptomics profile, was called the ERA® and nowadays is available as a diagnostic method for ARTs.

From this concept, the transcriptomic stratification of uterine receptivity has emerged, with this transcriptomic knowledge generating a new taxonomy of the WOI. Under this approach, the WOI may be understood as including different transcriptomic sub-signatures associated with different clinical outcomes related to menstrual cycle timing [15, 16]. The innovation of this procedure was to supervise transcriptomic predictors using as reference transcriptomic patterns as a new taxonomy for the WOI (Figure 4.4B). The clinical follow-up has distinguished between an optimal receptive profile with the best ongoing pregnancy rates and a late receptive sub-signature with a potential risk of biochemical pregnancies.

From the perspective of experimental design, researchers who study the endometrium have used menstrual cycle days and hormonal references to define groups and perform statistical comparisons [17, 11, 18]. In these studies, the LH peak was the reference, and classically LH+2 was the standard for pre-receptivity and LH+7 for receptivity [11]. Under this new transcriptomic stratification insight, the menstrual cycle samples are not grouped related to any physiological definition: after an unsupervised learning, samples are grouped depending on the gene expression profile and cluster defined previously [16].

Recently, a gene expression signature with predictive value for RIF has been described. Koot's signature used transcriptomic predictors and defined the WOI using LH measurements as the gold standard for timing (post-LH day 5 to post-LH day 8). The signature discovery process removed variations due to the WOI displacements, detecting a predictive pathological signature for RIF [18].

The Diaz-Gimeno signature and the Koot signature are essentially different from the design point of view, and only one gene is common to both. What remains unclear is whether both signatures are predicting similar or different types of RIF. However, evidence points to at least two main causes of RIF: WOI displacements and a heterogeneous transcriptomic disruption represented by Koot signatures [15].

The menstrual cycle timing context and its variations are a clue for evaluating endometrial receptivity in infertility. However, transcriptomic menstrual cycle timing is a confounding variable that should be controlled for distinguishing clearly between different RIF causes. Under this concept, RIF will be considered as a symptom and a new era in RIF taxonomy based on these genomic medicine approaches is under development and will provide a source of knowledge for precision medicine regarding the endometrial factor.

4.8　Clinical Application of the Endometrial Transcriptome

The ERA® is a commercially available endometrial analysis that includes the endometrial transcriptome as the basis of endometrial factor evaluation. This innovative tool identifies the endometrial dating transcriptomic signature coupled with a transcriptomic predictor capable of diagnosing an optimal receptive endometrium in terms of the best ongoing pregnancy rate.

The ERA enables detection of WOI displacements, detecting the WOI sub-signatures accurately identifying the optimal receptive period of an individual woman. This information can be used to personalize the progesterone administration days in HRT to promote the optimal endometrial profile and personalize the embryo transfer day, thus increasing live birth rates (Ruiz-Alonso et al., 2013b, 20).

The WOI is accepted as routinely located seven days after the LH surge in natural cycles or after five days of progesterone treatment previously primed with oestradiol in HRT cycles

(Figure 4.3). At that time, an endometrial biopsy is collected from any part of the uterine cavity in a previous cycle of embryo transfer. The expression profile is then processed in the ERA computational predictor to be classified into receptive or non-receptive status, which includes different WOI sub-signatures providing the accurate progesterone timing needed to induce the optimal receptivity (Figure 4.2). Although most patients were receptive during that time, clinical data obtained in 2,455 patients indicated that 25 per cent were non-receptive. Most of them had a delayed WOI (80 per cent), although in 20 per cent they had an advanced WOI [21].

Since the transcriptomic profile is determined in the previous cycle to that of embryo transfer, the consistency of the diagnosis in subsequent cycles has been also evaluated. A pilot study was performed with seven fertile patients biopsied twice in separate cycles. The similarity of the ERA expression pattern and the diagnoses in both samples were consistent even 29–40 months later. This clearly demonstrated that endometrium transcriptomic profiles do not change substantially between cycles within a single woman, in whom the hormonal treatment is the same [13].

Embryo transfer in patients with a displaced WOI suffers from asynchrony between the embryo and endometrium, decreasing the implantation rates and the ongoing pregnancies under these circumstances [20]. The diagnosis of the personalized WOI (pWOI) provides a personalized concept that guarantees that embryo transfer is being performed when the endometrium is 'ready to be implanted' by the embryo. This procedure enables matching of the embryo state (day 3 or day 5 blastocyst) with an optimal WOI by transferring at the specific recommended day.

On the other hand, the Diaz-Gimeno signature has been used as gold standard signature in research for the optimal endometrial receptivity status. The ERA transcriptome has been analysed in the effect of clinical treatments in endometrial preparation [22] and in pathological conditions as endometriosis [23] or obesity [24]. Table 4.1B summarizes the studies that have used ERA for determining endometrial status.

However, while this signature has been demonstrated as a powerful endometrial WOI biomarker with clinical applications, the pathological predictive value remains unclear.

4.9 Conclusion and Future Directions

Complex infertility traits such as implantation will be the most benefited in the era of precision medicine. Genomic medicine approaches have just arrived for endometrial factor evaluation. Transcriptomics predictors have revolutionized the endometrial factor evaluation in ART. The ERA test is a clear proof of concept in the infertility work-up, enabling a personalized embryo transfer that increases the rates of a successful embryo implantation and ongoing pregnancy. In the next years, other transcriptomic signatures will define other RIF causes, redefining the taxonomy of this infertility. Other promising genomic medicine approaches are not introduced yet in the reproductive field, but should in time provide new insights to underpin clinical practice.

Genomic differences between endometrial disorders leading to subfertility and the functional relationship between them, along with information of genetic variant profiles related to the regulation of the menstrual cycle [25], are examples of the promising discoveries that will improve the treatment of RIF and other subfertilities in the next years leading us to 'endometrial factor' causes.

References

1. Wilcox AJ, Baird DD, Weinberg CR. Time of implantation of the conceptus and loss of pregnancy. *N Engl J Med* 1999; **340**:1796–1799.

2. Feero WG, Guttmacher AE, Collins FS. Genomic Medicine – an updated primer. *N Engl J Med* 2010; **362(21)**:2001–2011.

3. Mirnezami R, Nicholson J, Darzi A. Preparing for Precision Medicine. *N Engl J Med* 2012; **366**:489–491.

4. Westerhoff HV, Palsson BO. The evolution of molecular biology into systems biology. 2004; **22**:1249–1252.

5. Goh K-I, Cusick ME, Valle D et al. The human disease network. *Proc Natl Acad Sci U S A* 2007; **104**:8685–8690.

6. Wang L, McLeod HL, Weinshilboum RM. Genomics and drug response. *N Engl J Med* 2011; **364**:1144–1153.

7. Gorini A, Pravettoni G. P5 Medicine: a plus for a personalized approach to oncology. *Nat Publ Gr* 2011; **2518**:2010–2011.

8. Van't Veer LJ, Dai H, Vijver MJ et al. Gene expression profiling predicts clinical outcome of breast cancer. *Nature* 2002; **415**:530–536.

9. Consortium M. The MicroArray Quality Control (MAQC)-II study of common practices for the development and validation of microarray-based predictive models. *Nat Biotechnol* 2010; **28**:827–838.

10. Vidal M, Cusick E, Barabási A. Interactome Networks and Human Disease. *Cell*. 2012; **144**:986–998.

11. Diaz-Gimeno P, Ruiz-Alonso M, Blesa D, Simón C. Transcriptomics of the human endometrium. *Int J Dev Biol* 2014; **58**:127–137.

12. Diaz-Gimeno P, Horcajadas JA, Martinez-Conejero JA et al. A genomic diagnostic tool for human endometrial receptivity based on the transcriptomic signature. *Fertil Steril* 2010; **27**: 50–60.

13. Diaz-Gimeno P, Ruiz-Alonso M, Blesa D et al. The accuracy and reproducibility of the endometrial receptivity array is superior to histology as a diagnostic method for endometrial receptivity. *Fertil Steril* 2013; **99**: 508–517.

14. Ruiz-Alonso M, Blesa D, Diaz-Gimeno P et al. The endometrial receptivity array for diagnosis and personalized embryo transfer as a treatment for patients with repeated implantation failure. *Fertil Steril* 2013; **100**:818–824.

15. Diaz-Gimeno P, Sebastian-Leon P, Remohí J, Garrido N, Pellicer A. New transcriptomic insight improves endometrial Recurrent Implantation Failure (RIF) diagnosis and distinguishes clearly between a displaced and a disrupted Window of Implantation (WOI). *ESRHE* 2017

16. Diaz-Gimeno P, Ruiz-Alonso M, Sebastian-Leon P et al. Window of implantation transcriptomic stratification reveals different endometrial sub-signatures associated to live birth and biochemical pregnancy. *Fertil Steril* in press

17. Altmäe S, Esteban FJ, Stavreus-Evers A et al. Guidelines for the design, analysis and interpretation of "omics" data: focus on human endometrium. *Hum Reprod Update* 2014; **20**:12–28.

18. Koot YEM, Hooff SR Van, Boomsma CM et al. An endometrial gene expression signature accurately predicts recurrent implantation failure after IVF. *Sci Rep* 2016; **6**:19411.

19. Díaz-Gimeno P. *Desarrollo De Una Herramienta Molecular Diagnóstica De La Receptividad Endometrial* 2011; Valencia University.

20. Ruiz-Alonso M, Galindo N, Pellicer A, Simón C. What a difference two days make: Personalized embryo transfer (pET) paradigm: A case report and pilot study. *Hum Reprod* 2014; **29**: 1244–1247.

21. Rincón A, Ruíz-Alonso M, Díaz-Gimeno P, Vilella F, Simón C. Endometrial Development and Gene Expression. In R. Farquharson & M. Stephenson, editors. *Early Pregnancy* 2017; pp. xi–xii. Cambridge: Cambridge University Press.

22. Bermejo A, Iglesias C, Ruiz-Alonso M et al. The impact of using the combined oral

contraceptive pill for cycle scheduling on gene expression related to endometrial receptivity. *Hum Reprod* 2014; **29**:1271–1278.

23. Garcia-Velasco JA, Fassbender A, Ruiz-Alonso M et al. Is endometrial receptivity transcriptomics affected in women with endometriosis? A pilot study. *Reprod Biomed Online* 2015; **31**:647–654.

24. Comstock IA, Diaz-Gimeno P, Cabanillas S et al. Does an increased body mass index affect endometrial gene expression patterns in infertile patients? A functional genomics analysis. *Fertil Steril* 2017; **107**:740–748.

25. Fung JN, Girling JE, Lukowski SW et al. The genetic regulation of transcription in human endometrial tissue. *Hum Reprod* 2017; **32**:1–12.

Effects of Superovulation on the Endometrium

Natalie Hannan and Jemma Evans

5.1 The Endometrium

The human endometrium is a highly complex and dynamic tissue that undergoes controlled cyclical remodelling and differentiation throughout reproductive life, regulated primarily by the ovarian steroid hormones, progesterone and oestrogen (Figure 5.1)[1]. The menstrual

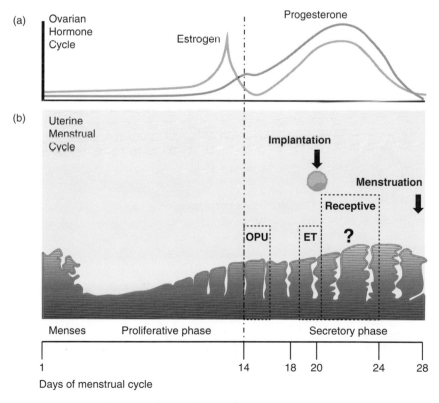

Figure 5.1 Human menstrual cycle. Endometrial remodelling across a standardized 28-day menstrual cycle is driven by changes in circulating levels of ovarian steroid hormones. The endometrium regenerates under the control of oestrogen and differentiates under the control of progesterone to produce an environment suitable for embryo implantation. In the absence of implantation, progesterone withdrawal accompanying corpus luteum regression leads to endometrial breakdown and menstruation. In an IVF cycle (boxed), hormonal stimulation of the ovaries can disturb endometrial receptivity. A: serum hormone levels; B: endometrial alterations. Box: the IVF situation. **ET**: embryo transfer; **IVF**: in vitro fertilization; **OPU**: ovum pickup

cycle can be divided into three main phases: menses (breakdown and degradation), proliferative (regeneration) and secretory (differentiation). The endometrium is composed of many different cell types: epithelial (luminal and glandular) cells, stromal cells, leukocytes and cells associated with blood vessels, including endothelial and perivascular cells (covered in detail, this volume, Chapter 1).

Proliferation of all endometrial cell types occurs during the follicular phase of the ovarian cycle [2]; during the secretory phase, cells cease proliferation and undergo post-ovulatory differentiation. At the end of a non-conception cycle, the demise of the corpus luteum causes the levels of progesterone (and oestrogen) to fall. The fall in progesterone initiates menstruation [1].

5.2 Endometrial Receptivity and Implantation

Endometrial remodelling is essential for transition from a hostile to a receptive state, to allow blastocyst attachment and trophoblast invasion. This receptive phase encompasses a short period of time spanning menstrual cycle days 20–24 (luteinizing hormone (LH)+ 7–LH+11) and is known as the 'window of implantation' [1].

A series of key morphological and functional changes are observed in the endometrium when preparing for implantation (covered in detail, this volume, Chapter 2). It is now well accepted that successful preparation of a receptive endometrium comprises the acquisition of adhesion ligands and the synchronized loss of inhibitory components that may prevent blastocyst attachment to the epithelium [2]. Therefore, the tightly controlled expression of

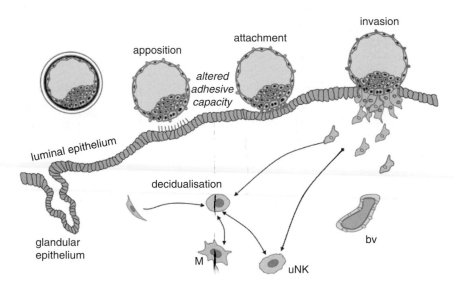

Figure 5.2 The developing pre-implantation embryo enters the uterine cavity as an unhatched blastocyst, and within the microenvironment of the uterine cavity, it hatches, becomes apposed to and then attaches to the endometrial luminal epithelium. Subsequently, the outer trophectoderm cells pass between the epithelial cells and invade through the basal lamina to enter a new environment of decidualizing stromal cells. The trophectoderm subsequently differentiates into a number of trophoblast types (cyto-, syncytio- and extravillous trophoblast), which variably secrete cytokines and other factors, further driving the decidualization of the stroma, recruitment of a specific population of leukocytes (particularly macrophages (M) and uterine natural killer (NK) cells) into the site. The extravillous trophoblast homes to maternal spiral arterioles throughout the decidua. Some of these eventually penetrate and remodel the vasculature to provide increased blood flow essential for pregnancy

adhesion and anti-adhesion proteins is essential for establishing a maternal-embryonic interaction.

Pregnancy success is dependent on a complex dialogue between the embryo and the maternal endometrium, initially dependent on secreted factors (both soluble and within extracellular vesicles) within the local microenvironment of the uterine cavity, but also includes subsequent interactions within the decidua (Figure 5.2). This early communication is optimal during the window of implantation. It is clear that alterations in the timing of endometrial development during each menstrual cycle or the quality of endometrial receptivity during this window are highly implicated in failures of IVF. This is highlighted by a study showing that 30 per cent of euploid single blastocyst transfers, in good prognosis patients, did not result in a pregnancy [3].

5.3   The Endometrium in Controlled Ovarian Stimulative Cycles

As described previously, in natural menstrual cycles in normo-ovulatory women, following post-menstrual repair, the endometrium regenerates during the proliferative phase (largely driven by rising oestrogen). Following ovulation and formation of the corpus luteum, progesterone begins to rise; coincidently the endometrium undergoes secretory transformation, progressively towards a state of receptivity whereby key changes in both endometrial epithelial and stromal cells occur, along with changes in the vasculature, extracellular matrix and leucocyte content of the tissue [4]. However, when superovulation is induced for oocyte harvesting with exogenous hormones (Figure 5.1), the endometrium is exposed to supraphysiological concentrations of oestrogen and progesterone, which can dramatically augment endometrial development, and thus the timing of endometrial receptivity [5]. Patients with high oestradiol concentrations produce significantly more oocytes and also have elevated progesterone concentrations. If pregnancy is achieved, the effect of elevated oestradiol can be far-reaching: for example, the risk for antepartum haemorrhage increases with increasing oocyte numbers and oestradiol concentrations [6].

Aberrant steroid hormone concentrations have been known for some time to detrimentally affect endometrial morphology and therefore receptivity (reviewed [7]). A systematic review and meta-analysis of pregnancy outcomes following precocious progesterone elevation on the day of human chorionic gonadotrophin (hCG) administration (0.08 ng/ml) demonstrated that a premature rise in progesterone is associated with reduced pregnancy rates in fresh embryo transfer cycles, but not in frozen/thawed or donor–recipient IVF cycles [8]. This suggests a detrimental impact on endometrial receptivity in stimulation cycles and highlights that a fine balance of steroid hormones is needed to confer endometrial receptivity. Disparities in endometrial tissue at the molecular level have been identified in genomic analyses of stimulated endometria from women with elevated progesterone concentrations (versus those with normal progesterone concentrations), sampled between hCG+7and hCG+8. Both miRNA and mRNA expressions were dysregulated in those with raised progesterone levels [7].

5.4   Histological, Transcriptomic and Proteomic Studies

Dramatic differences between the normal cycling endometrium and endometrium from superovulation cycles have been demonstrated at the histological, transcriptomic and proteomic levels in both the tissue and the intrauterine environment. Taken together, these data provide strong evidence that endometrial receptivity is disturbed with superovulation protocols and thus likely limits the success of fresh embryo transfer.

Histologically, an advancement in endometrial dating of ≥3 days (as assessed by highly experienced pathologists using Noyes' criteria for endometrial dating) in women stimulated with either a GnRH agonist or a GnRH antagonist protocol was associated with a complete failure to achieve pregnancy/implantation [7]. However, a more recent comprehensive histological/immunohistochemical study suggests that the absence of receptivity is more complicated than mere developmental advancement, and that a complex lack of synchrony of development between the different cellular and structural compartments of the endometrium results from ovarian stimulation protocols [9]. This comprehensive study of endometrial histology was performed in five groups of women at LH/hCG+2. These were: (1) GnRH agonist-treated oocyte donors; (2) GnRH agonist-treated women who subsequently failed to become pregnant following fresh embryo transfer (within the same cycle); (3) GnRH agonist-treated women who became pregnant following fresh embryo transfer; (4) GnRH antagonist-treated women with unsuccessful fresh embryo transfer; and (5) normal fertile women (LH+2) as the comparison group. Major alterations in endometrial histology following stimulation for multi-follicular development were observed in this study (Figure 5.3). Changes in endometrial histology, leukocyte subtype and number, progesterone receptor expression and vascular markers were assessed and scored for individual cellular compartments to determine endometrial perturbations. Specifically, endometrial glandular and luminal epithelium, stroma and vasculature in endometrium from women undergoing IVF were assessed in tissues at hCG+2 in comparison to normal cycling women at LH+2. Women treated with GnRH agonist or GnRH antagonist protocols who did not become pregnant within the same cycle following embryo transfer displayed significantly altered endometrial histology based on eight different parameters (Figure 5.3). The alterations in endometrial histology did not appear to be related to their infertility as fertile oocyte donors receiving the GnRH agonist protocol displayed a similar degree of endometrial changes. Most importantly, women who became pregnant following ovarian stimulation and embryo transfer displayed significantly fewer perturbed histological alterations than did the women who failed to become pregnant, emphasizing that the extent of endometrial disturbance impacted successful implantation [9]. However, it is important to note that while these women with 'less' perturbed endometrium achieved a pregnancy, the obstetric and perinatal outcomes for these pregnancies were not known. Further work is needed to compare an 'endometrial disturbance index' with birth and longer-term outcomes. Indeed, a recent study has identified that supraphysiological oestradiol is a predictor for low birthweight in full-term singleton births from fresh embryo transfer cycles [10].

Other data support endometrial advancement as a major reason for failure to establish a viable pregnancy. In natural pregnancies, implantation that has occurred late in the menstrual cycle (as determined by ultrasensitive hCG detection in urine) is associated with early pregnancy loss [11]. 'Advanced' endometrial maturation on the day of oocyte retrieval has also been characterized by altered gene expression [7]; 1337 genes reported as elevated and 1213 genes down-regulated in significantly advanced (≥3 days) endometria. Indeed, many transcriptomic profiling studies of the stimulated endometrium have revealed alterations in gene expression in the endometrium taken between hCG+2 and hCG+7 compared with the natural cycle [7], although specific gene changes are not consistent between studies. Furthermore, in a tightly controlled cohort using cycle-matched endometrial samples, taken from the same women at LH+7 in non-stimulated cycles and hCG+7 in a subsequent stimulated cycle, 281 genes were elevated and 277 down-regulated at hCG+7 [12]. Importantly, of the identified genes, those with known roles in implantation, including

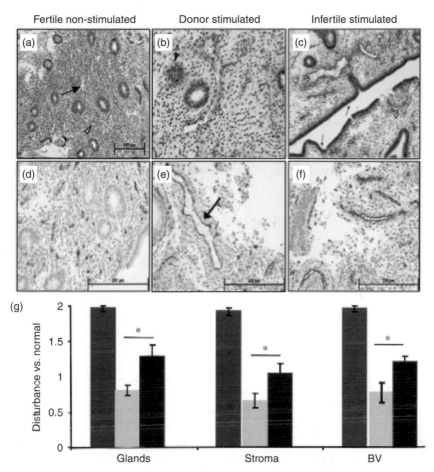

Figure 5.3 A–C. Haematoxylin and eosin-stained endometrial sections. In non-stimulated endometrium from fertile women collected at LH+2 (**A**), the glands are small and straight with only very early signs of secretory changes. The stroma is compact with minor signs of oedema (arrow), and blood vessels are few and small (open arrow head). **B.** In stimulated (GnRH agonist; hCG+2) endometrium from fertile donors, staining reveals the presence of more abundant, larger vessels in the stroma surrounding the glands (open arrow head); these glands have signs of more advanced cycle stage subnuclear vacuole formation (closed arrow head). (**C**) Stimulated endometria from infertile women (GnRH agonist; hCG+2) who did not subsequently become pregnant show perturbed expanded oedematous stroma, with enlarged sub-epithelial (arrows indicate luminal epithelium) blood vessels filled with red blood cells (open arrow heads), indicating the fragile state of the tissue.

 D–F. The vessels are better visualized by immunostaining for the vascular marker CD34. (**D**) Blood vessels within the endometria of fertile women at LH+2 were generally small and compact. (**E**) Endometria from hormonally stimulated fertile women (GnRH agonist; hCG+2) revealed a mixture of small blood vessels and grossly enlarged blood vessels (arrow). (**F**) Examination of endometria from stimulated infertile women (GnRH antagonist; hCG+2) displayed a varied and perturbed vascular network. (**G**) Alterations in the endometrium in stimulation cycles on hCG+2. Semi-quantitative assessment of eight features of endometrial morphology (glandular and luminal epithelium, stroma and vasculature, including specific immunohistochemical markers from data described in Evans et al., 2012) for each tissue type and normalized to those of control samples. Blue bar: non-stimulated fertile women, LH+2; grey bar: infertile, agonist (no pregnancy); black bar: infertile, agonist (pregnant)

leukaemia inhibitory factor (LIF) and glycodelin, were down-regulated at hCG+7. In addition, the Macklon group [13] has shown a significant elevation in Dickkopf-related protein 1 (DKK-1), produced by decidualized endometrial stromal cells, in the endometrium of women treated with GnRH antagonist, strongly suggesting advanced development at hCG+2, particularly since decidual stromal cells (a key feature of the late and not early secretory endometrium) have been observed in some stimulated tissues at this time [9].

Genomic analyses have revealed significant alterations in a host of CCL- and CXCL-chemokines during the pre-receptive to receptive transition and in stimulated endometrial tissues. These alterations are reinforced by analysis of uterine cavity fluid from a mixed GnRH agonist/GnRH antagonist-stimulated population [14], which revealed higher concentrations of CCL- and CXCL-chemokines secreted from the endometrium into the uterine cavity, including interleukin (IL)-1β, IL-5, IL-10, IL-12, eotaxin, DKK-1 and heparin-binding epidermal growth factor at hCG+6, compared with concentrations in normally fertile women at LH+6. Such changes in inflammatory chemokine production by the stimulated endometrium may reflect a more inflamed tissue, and in the case of elevated DKK-1 also a more advanced endometrium (as discussed above). Recent data suggest that the presence of an inflamed environment within the endometrium is detrimental to implantation. Indeed, Evans et al. [9] demonstrated that not only are leukocyte numbers elevated within stimulated endometrium but, more importantly, activated leucocytes, including abundant degranulating neutrophils, classically associated with the inflammatory milieu at menstruation, were present in the stimulated endometrium of women who did not become pregnant. Thus, local inflammation in combination with endometrial advancement is likely to contribute to the deficient receptivity and hence failure of implantation in these women.

Vast enlargement of blood vessels is also a clear feature of endometrium in both agonist- and antagonist-treated women on hCG+2 [9] (Figure 5.3). In particular, very large vessels are clearly visible immediately below the endometrial surface in agonist-treated women who failed to become pregnant following fresh embryo transfer (Figure 5.3). Although the molecular mechanisms underpinning these vascular changes are not yet defined, they are in accordance with the increase in vascular permeability seen in ovarian hyper-stimulation syndrome (OHSS). The hCG, administered to stimulate ovulation, is a likely protagonist, yet blastocyst-secreted hCG can act acutely on the endometrium in conception cycles, stimulating epithelial cell production of a number of mediators, including vascular endothelial growth factor A and fibroblast growth factor 2 (FGF2), both potent angiogenic factors [15,16]. Thus, the use of hCG for ovarian stimulation may have additional detrimental actions on the endometrium in an IVF cycle.

5.5 Human Chorionic Gonadotrophin

The hCG gene is transcribed by the embryo from the eight-cell stage, and hCG protein is secreted by the embryo from the late blastocyst stage, approximately seven to eight days after fertilization. The 'classic' role of hCG is considered to be its luteotrophic function in maintaining the corpus luteum, and thus progesterone production in the early stages of pregnancy. Indeed, this action is essential for pregnancy establishment.

Due to its structural similarities to LH and its ability to occupy the same receptor, the LH/CG receptor, hCG is widely used in IVF to mimic the mid-cycle LH surge. However, significant differences exist in the half-lives of these ligands; while that of LH is short, ~60 min, hCG has a much longer half-life of >24 h. It has been estimated that following a bolus of 10,000 IU hCG, a dose commonly used to stimulate ovulation, hCG levels in serum remain elevated for >5 days [17]. It is therefore likely that prolonged stimulation of the LH/hCG receptor will have detrimental effects both on ovarian function in the luteal phase and on the endometrium [7].

A non-gonadotropic role for hCG was first demonstrated by Licht et al. [18]; the infusion of hCG directly into the uterine cavity of women revealed profound changes in endometrial secretions. Specifically, inhibition of prolactin, insulin-like growth factor-binding protein-1 (IGFBP-1) and macrophage colony-stimulating factor (M-CSF), as well as biphasic regulation of vascular endothelial growth factor (VEGF), was identified with direct hCG exposure. Subsequent studies in which hCG was similarly infused into the uterine cavity of baboons [19], and in which hCG was added to primary human endometrial epithelial cells in vitro [16, 20], validated and extended these findings, demonstrating that hCG enhances the expression and secretion of factors considered key to implantation, including LIF, prokineticin-1, IL-6, IL-11, granulocyte-macrophage colony-stimulating factor (GMCSF), VEGF, fibroblast growth factor 2 (FGF2) and CXCL10. Therefore, it is likely that during the normal peri-implantation period in a conception cycle, blastocyst-derived hCG can enhance endometrial receptivity.

In the in vitro experimental setting, these 'pro-implantation' factors were induced in endometrial epithelial cells by only a short duration of exposure to hCG in culture (as would be the case with the presence of a peri-implantation blastocyst). However, in the baboon model, when hCG was continuously infused into the uterine cavity for five days, the endometrial LH-CG receptor (R), through which hCG exerts its action, was down-regulated [19,21]. This indicated that the endometrium becomes less responsive to hCG upon prolonged exposure, due to receptor down-regulation. Indeed, this phenomenon was first described in gonadal tissues more than 30 years ago [7].

LH-CGR down-regulation has recently been confirmed in human endometrial biopsies taken two days after the hCG trigger (hCG+2). The subjects were undergoing IVF using either GnRH agonist or GnRH antagonist stimulation protocols followed by triggering with a single bolus of recombinant hCG (rhCG; 250 μg) [22]. The endometrial epithelial LH-CGR was significantly down-regulated in the IVF endometria exposed to hCG in comparison with tissue taken at LH+2 from normally cycling, age-matched women of known fertility. Subsequent functional cell culture studies confirmed the importance of receptor down-regulation on embryonic–endometrial crosstalk for implantation. Following pre-exposure to hCG, mimicking the timing of exposure in an IVF cycle (Figure 5.4), endometrial epithelial cells could no longer mount a functional implantation response to a blastocyst. The LHCG-R was down-regulated, and thus intracellular signalling (ERK 1/2 phosphorylation) could not be activated, and the cells could not adhere to trophoblast-like extracellular matrices and could not relax intercellular tight junctions [22]: all of these are endometrial functions normally regulated by hCG. These data suggest that precocious exposure of the endometrium to hCG, outside the timing of the window of implantation, down-regulates the endometrial epithelial LHCG-R, thus increasing the likelihood that the endometrium may be poorly responsive to the subsequent blastocyst-derived hCG that would normally promote endometrial changes to enhance receptivity. These effects are summarized diagrammatically in Figure 5.4.

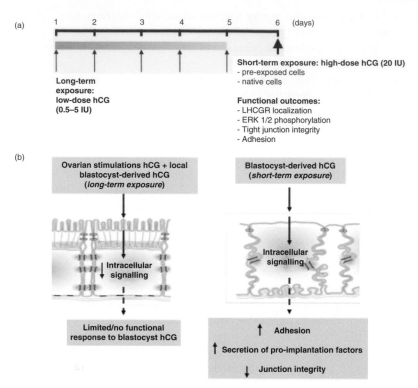

Figure 5.4 Schematic summarizing of experimentally proven alterations in the response of the endometrium to either blastocyst hCG within a normal pregnancy or within a cycle in which hCG has been used to induce ovulation. **A.** Endometrial epithelial cells were treated with a low dose of hCG (0.5–5 IU) each day for five days (arrows). Both cells pre-exposed to hCG and naïve cells (never been exposed to hCG) were then treated with 20 IU hCG to mimic that secreted by the incoming blastocyst in a conception cycle and functional outcomes were examined. **B.** In cells pre-exposed to low doses of hCG, 20 IU hCG could not mediate signalling, relaxation of tight junctions or adhesiveness. In these pre-exposed cells, the LHCG-R was down-regulated, suggesting the cells were refractory to hCG. In naïve cells exposed to the dose of hCG mimicking endometrial exposure to blastocyst-secreted hCG for the first time as experienced in a normal conception cycle, 20IU hCG enhanced ERK1/2 phosphorylation, relaxation of intercellular tight junctions and adhesiveness of endometrial epithelial cells to trophoblast-like extracellular matrices, all of which are important features of the epithelium associated with successful implantation. (From [7])

5.6 The Stimulated Endometrium with Respect to Pregnancy Success: Clinical Implications and Lessons from Non-Human Models

The LH/CG-R is also down-regulated after the spontaneous LH surge [23]. It may be that the observed LHCG-R down-regulation in the endometrium on hCG+2 relative to LH+2 is only transient, and that the receptor recovers by the time implantation occurs five days later. It is difficult to test in women (in vivo) what happens to the receptor levels or whether there is activation of down-stream pathways in the presence of a blastocyst. However, in pseudo-pregnant rats, ovarian LH/CG-R mRNA was suppressed for 48 h after a large bolus of hCG, but it recovered to control levels in rats after 53 h [24]. This study, however, did not investigate protein levels of the receptor, nor its functionality. Further, rats and mice have very short oestrous cycles (4–5 days) and different endometrial responses to stimuli, compared with the much longer cycles (approximately 28 days) in women. In baboons, a primate species also with 28-day menstrual cycles, administration of hCG for 5–6 days following ovulation showed reduced endometrial epithelial LH/CG-R protein in endometrial tissue obtained 6 days later [21]. Recent in vivo evidence in women supports this, demonstrating longer-lasting endometrial changes in response to hCG. A study comparing a traditional hCG ovulation trigger followed by luteal phase progesterone versus a GnRH agonist trigger followed by either (1) oestrogen and progesterone or (2) recombinant LH combined with oestrogen and progesterone found that the endometrial gene expression profiles were significantly different seven days after the hCG trigger, which coincides with the window of implantation [25]. Interestingly, ADAMTS8, a proteinase with potent anti-angiogenic properties, was up-regulated in the hCG ovulation trigger group at hCG+7 compared with those receiving the GnRH trigger, demonstrating that the effects of hCG used for ovulation are likely perpetuated, mediating detrimental effects on the endometrium within the same stimulation cycle. Thus, it is likely that the sixfold higher expression of ADAMTS8 in endometria exposed to recombinant hCG plays a role in initiating abnormal placentation, and therefore ultimately results in some of the adverse perinatal outcomes associated with fresh embryo transfers.

Despite substantial differences in implantation between species, rodents can provide functional models for studies that are not possible in women. Embryo transfer studies in rodents (in which embryos were transferred to recipient female mice that had undergone ovarian stimulation) showed a significant decrease in successful implantation compared with embryo transfer to control (not stimulated) recipients, again indicative of an effect of ovarian stimulation protocols on endometrial receptivity. More recent molecular studies in a rat ovarian stimulation model have further defined these changes, including (1) altered uterine expression of TGF-β1 and -β2 and (2) decreased β3 integrin and VEGF, in agreement with human data.

In conclusion, there is now considerable scientific and clinical evidence of major disturbances to the human endometrium due to current ovarian stimulation protocols for women undergoing ART. This appears to be irrespective of whether the woman has unexplained infertility or is fertile. Furthermore, the perturbations observed are greater in women who fail to become pregnant in the same cycle (following stimulation), indicating a reason for the failure. Increasing evidence is also emerging that pregnancies that occur in the same cycle as stimulation have poorer obstetric and perinatal outcomes. We propose that the disturbed endometrial transformation in preparation for pregnancy observed with ovarian stimulation renders the endometrium poorly or non-receptive for embryo implantation, indicating that either modification of protocols or transfer of frozen embryos into natural cycles may optimize outcomes for infertile couples and improve the quality of placentation and thus the resultant pregnancy.

References

1. Evans J, Salamonsen LA, Winship A et al. Fertile ground: human endometrial programming and lessons in health and disease. *Nat Rev Endocrinol* 2016; 12: 654–67.

2. Aplin JD, Ruane PT. Embryo-epithelium interactions during implantation at a glance. *J Cell Sci* 2017; 130:15–22.

3. Yang Z, Liu J, Collins GS et al. Selection of single blastocysts for fresh transfer via standard morphology assessment alone and with array CGH for good prognosis IVF patients: results from a randomized pilot study. *Mol Cytogenet* 2012; 5:24.

4. Maybin JA, Critchley HO. Menstrual physiology: implications for endometrial pathology and beyond. *Hum Reprod Update* 2015; 21:748–61.

5. Fauser BC, Devroey P. Reproductive biology and IVF: ovarian stimulation and luteal phase consequences. *Trends Endocrinol Metab* 2003; 14:236–42.

6. Healy DL, Breheny S, Halliday J et al. Prevalence and risk factors for obstetric haemorrhage in 6730 singleton births after assisted reproductive technology in Victoria Australia. *Hum Reprod* 2010; 25: 265–74.

7. Evans J, Hannan NJ, Edgell TA et al. Fresh versus frozen embryo transfer: backing clinical decisions with scientific and clinical evidence. *Hum Reprod Update* 2014; 20:808–21.

8. Venetis CA, Kolibianakis EM, Bosdou JK, Tarlatzis BC. Progesterone elevation and probability of pregnancy after IVF: a systematic review and meta-analysis of over 60 000 cycles. *Hum Reprod Update* 2013; 19:433–57.

9. Evans J, Hannan NJ, Hincks C, Rombauts LJ, Salamonsen LA. Defective soil for a fertile seed? Altered endometrial development is detrimental to pregnancy success. *PLoS One* 2012; 7:e53098.

10. Pereira N, Elias RT, Christos PJ et al. Supraphysiologic estradiol is an independent predictor of low birth weight in full-term singletons born after fresh embryo transfer. *Hum Reprod* 2017; 32: 1410–17.

11. Wilcox AJ, Baird DD, Weinberg CR. Time of implantation of the conceptus and loss of pregnancy. *N Engl J Med* 1999; 340: 1796–9.

12. Horcajadas JA, Riesewijk A, Polman J et al. Effect of controlled ovarian hyperstimulation in IVF on endometrial gene expression profiles. *Mol Hum Reprod* 2005; 11:195–205.

13. Macklon NS, van der Gaast MH, Hamilton A, Fauser BC, Giudice LC. The impact of ovarian stimulation with recombinant FSH in combination with GnRH antagonist on the endometrial transcriptome in the window of implantation. *Reprod Sci* 2008; 15:357–65.

14. Boomsma CM, Kavelaars A, Eijkemans MJ et al. Ovarian stimulation for in vitro fertilization alters the intrauterine cytokine, chemokine, and growth factor milieu encountered by the embryo. *Fertil Steril* 2010; 94:1764–8.

15. Licht P, Fluhr H, Neuwinger J, Wallwiener D, Wildt L. Is human chorionic gonadotropin directly involved in the regulation of human implantation? *Mol Cell Endocrinol* 2007; 269:85–92.

16. Paiva P, Hannan NJ, Hincks C et al. Human chorionic gonadotrophin regulates FGF2 and other cytokines produced by human endometrial epithelial cells, providing a mechanism for enhancing endometrial receptivity. *Hum Reprod* 2011; 26:1153–62.

17. Chan CC, Ng EH, Chan MM et al. Bioavailability of hCG after intramuscular or subcutaneous injection in obese and non-obese women. *Hum Reprod* 2003; 18: 2294–7.

18. Licht P, Losch A, Dittrich R et al. Novel insights into human endometrial paracrinology and embryo-maternal communication by intrauterine microdialysis. *Hum Reprod Update* 1998; 4: 532–8.

19. Sherwin JR, Sharkey AM, Cameo P et al. Identification of novel genes regulated by chorionic gonadotropin in baboon endometrium during the window of implantation. *Endocrinology* 2007; 148: 618–26.

20. Evans J, Catalano RD, Brown P et al. Prokineticin 1 mediates fetal-maternal dialogue regulating endometrial leukemia inhibitory factor. *FASEB J* 2009; 23: 2165–75.

21. Cameo P, Szmidt M, Strakova Z et al. Decidualization regulates the expression of the endometrial chorionic gonadotropin receptor in the primate. *Biol Reprod* 2006; 75:681–9.

22. Evans J, Salamonsen LA. Too much of a good thing? Experimental evidence suggests prolonged exposure to hCG is

detrimental to endometrial receptivity. *Hum Reprod* 2013; 28:1610–9.

23. Menon KM, Menon B. Structure, function and regulation of gonadotropin receptors – a perspective. *Mol Cell Endocrinol* 2012; 356:88–97.

24. Harada M, Peegel H, Menon KM. Expression of vascular endothelial growth factor A during ligand-induced down-regulation of luteinizing hormone receptor in the ovary. *Mol Cell Endocrinol* 2010; 328:28–33.

25. Bermejo A, Iglesias C, Ruiz-Alonso M et al. The impact of using the combined oral contraceptive pill for cycle scheduling on gene expression related to endometrial receptivity. *Hum Reprod* 2014; 29:1271–8.

Chapter

6

Screening the Uterine Microbiome Prior to Embryo Transfer

Inmaculada Moreno and Carlos Simon

6.1 Introduction

The human microbiome is composed of all the microorganisms (archaea, bacteria, eukaryotes and viruses) inhabiting the human body and their genomes. The Human Microbiome Project (HMP) has characterized the core microbiome of different body sites (oral, respiratory, gastrointestinal and urogenital tracts, and skin) to understand its role in human health and disease [1]. These studies have revealed that up to 100 trillion microbes live in association with the cells in the human body, contributing 150 times more functional microbial DNA than human genes [2]. From all the microorganisms inhabiting the human body, the main interest has been focused on bacteria, concentrating the majority of the studies on human microbiome. A balanced microbiome provides fundamental biological functions to the host which include digestion, production of essential compounds as well as training of the immune system, while alterations of the microbiome associate with specific diseases and other pathological states (reviewed in [2]).

6.1.1 Technical Assessment of the Microbiome

The analysis of the bacteria present in biological samples has been traditionally undertaken by isolation, growth and count of colony forming units under selective media and conditions. However, it is now known that up to 80 per cent of the bacteria colonizing the human body do not grow under standard in vitro culture conditions. This means that using culture-dependent techniques may yield results in which the diversity of the sample would be underestimated, generating misleading conclusions about the physiologic or pathologic roles of the bacterial community in each specific body site [3]. During the last decade, the methods for the analysis of the bacterial communities present in any given sample have changed from the classical microbiological culture to molecular techniques including fingerprint polymerase chain reaction (PCR), microarrays, as well as targeted and whole genome sequencing (Figure 6.1). These molecular methods not only enable the identification of difficult to culture bacteria but also provide the information about the proportions in which each individual bacterium was present in the initial sample. Targeted detection of bacteria, regardless of the method used, PCR, microarray or next-generation sequencing (NGS) is based on the previous knowledge of bacterial gene sequences and results are inferred by comparison of the resulting data to closest bacteria included in existent databases. Thus, no discovery of new bacterial species or strains is possible by using these methods. Concretely, the bacterial gene encoding for the 16S ribosomal RNA has been widely used in the detection of bacterial populations within samples. This gene has the distinctive feature of containing nine hypervariable regions (V1–V9) which have diverged

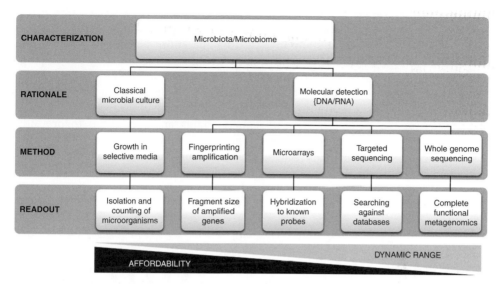

Figure 6.1 Scheme of the different techniques to characterize the microbiome
Source: Adapted from *Fertility and Sterility*, 104(6), Mor A, Driggers PH and Segars JH, Molecular characterization of the human microbiome from a reproductive perspective, 1344–1350, Copyright 2015, with permission from Elsevier.

with evolution to show species-specific DNA sequences flanked by highly conserved regions. Then, using specific primers designed against the variable regions of the 16S for specific bacteria of interest will allow the amplification by fingerprinting PCR and detection of the bacteria. On the other hand, the use of primers designed against the conserved regions of this gene allows the enrichment and sequencing of the variable regions of every bacterium contained in the sample, permitting the rapid and accurate taxonomic classification based on known 16S databases [3]. This evolution has been promoted by the technical advances in massive parallel sequencing along with the decrease in the cost of such analysis. Finally, the most advanced method for the metagenomic analysis of the microbiome consists in the unbiased sequencing of DNA (or whole genome sequencing) and subsequent assembling to bacterial genomes. Because this strategy is not restricted to the 16S rRNA gene, the results not only reveal the bacterial population colonizing a sample but also provide information about the functional impact of the genes detected in the sample and the potential interaction of the bacterial community with the host. However, comprehensive molecular detection of microbiomes presents some limitations due to the complexity and heterogeneity of the microbes. The first challenge in culture-independent techniques concerns the efficient release of representative high-quality DNA from bacteria with different cell wall and membrane thickness. Also, metagenomics-driven techniques do not discriminate between live or dead bacteria, so strict controls should be included in microbiome experiments to discard potential contaminations [2].

6.2 The Microbiome of the Female Reproductive Tract

Around 9 per cent of the total bacteria colonizing the human body reside in the female urogenital tract. While the most prevalent bacteria identified in the reproductive tract of voluntary healthy women are *Lactobacilli*, which account for up to 85–90 per cent of abundance in the average population, other bacterial genera as *Prevotella, Gardnerella, Atopobium, Sneathia, Bifidobacterium, Megasphera* and *Anaerococcus* have also been commonly identified [4]. A recent study investigating the entire female reproductive tract microbiome has been conducted in women undergoing total hysterectomy and salpingo-oopherectomy [5]. This study has compared the bacterial communities simultaneously present in the vagina, cervix, uterus, fallopian tubes and ovaries of ten individuals (Figure 6.2). The results of this study confirm that bacterial colonization of the reproductive tract is not restricted to the lower genital tract, namely vagina and cervix, but to previously considered sterile organs as the endometrium, fallopian tubes and ovaries. Also, although the study presents some limitations related to the low sample size and the characteristics of the patients recruited in the study (age, gynaecological condition, surgical procedure, menopausal status, etc.), this study shows for the first time that significant differences can

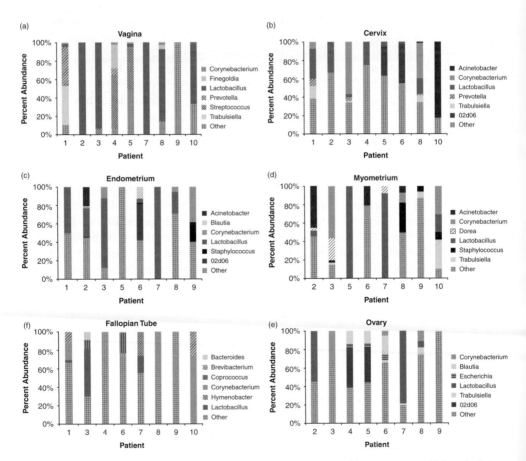

Figure 6.2 Reproductive tract microbiome in ten women undergoing a total hysterectomy and bilateral salpingo-oopherectomy. Distribution of the most common bacterial genera in different body sites: vagina, cervix, endometrium, myometrium, fallopian tubes and ovaries. Scheme of the different techniques to characterize the microbiome

Source: Reprinted from *Fertility and Sterility*, 107(3), Miles SM, Hardy BL and Merrell DS, Investigation of the microbiota of the reproductive tract in women undergoing a total hysterectomy and bilateral salpingo-oopherectomy, 813–820, Copyright 2017, with permission from Elsevier.

be found in the microbial profiles, at the genus or species level, of different body sites within the female reproductive tract [5].

6.2.1 The Lower Genital Tract Microbiome

Most of the current knowledge on the reproductive tract microbiome comes from the analysis of vaginal samples. It is well accepted that the vaginal microbiota of reproductive-age women is mainly composed of bacteria from the *Lactobacillus* genus, although some other bacterial genera as *Atopobium, Gardnerella, Prevotella, Sneathia* and others can also populate the vagina in physiological conditions. The vaginal microbiome has been classified into five major groups or community state types (CSTs) based on the most dominant bacteria present in such samples. Following this nomenclature, CST-I, -II, -III and -V, dominated by *L. crispatus, L. gasserii, L. iners* and *L. jensenii*, respectively, have been associated with vaginal health, while CST-IV, characterized by displacement of *Lactobacilli* for anaerobic bacteria often correlates with bacterial vaginosis [6]. Nonetheless, the presence of dysbiotic species does not imply a pathological state, as the vaginal microbiome is highly variable depending on several factors as age, ethnicity, phase of the menstrual cycle, oestrogen levels, sexual activity or hygiene [7] reaching a higher stability during normal pregnancy [8]. While vaginal microbiomes dominated by *Lactobacillus* (CST-I, -II, -III and -V) have been classically associated with genital health, the characteristic that increased vaginal diversity of CST-IV is a predisposing factor for sexually transmitted infections, human papillomavirus, human immunodeficiency virus type 1 and other gynaecological infections, as well as pregnancy complications [9].

6.2.2 The Upper Genital Tract Microbiome

Challenging the pre-existing dogma of a sterile onset of life, several studies to date have started to uncover the microbiota of the organs forming the upper genital tract. Interestingly, the average amount of bacteria present in the upper genital tract are 100 to 10,000 times lower than that on the vagina, consistent with the external location of the vagina [10]. Lately, an active microbiome has been reported in ovaries and fallopian tubes of reproductive-age women. It has been reported that colonization of the follicular environment by *Lactobacillus* spp. yield improved reproductive outcomes than colonization by other genera such as *Propionibacterium* or *Actinomyces*, suggesting a functional role for these bacteria in the ovarian niche [11]. In this regard, shifts in the physiological microbiota in the ovary could lead to alterations in follicle development, premature ovarian failure and polycystic ovarian syndrome, among other pathologies [5].

6.3 The Uterine Microbiome

Isolation of bacteria by culture of endometrial samples has been classically linked to reproductive tract infections. This association is supported by studies in which polymicrobial biofilms including *Gardnerella vaginalis* have been found in the endometrium and fallopian tubes of patients diagnosed with bacterial vaginosis [12]. However, several studies to date have demonstrated the existence of bacteria in the uterine cavity in non-pathological conditions. In 2015, Mitchell and collaborators compared the microbiota of lower and upper genital tract of 58 women undergoing hysterectomy for benign conditions. By analysing the 16S rRNA gene content by quantitative PCR for a set of 12 bacterial taxa, they identified bacteria in 95 per cent of the endometrial analysed samples. The presence of bacteria in the endometrium did not associate with any sign or inflammation or the diagnosis of bacterial vaginosis. Interestingly, this study demonstrated that vaginal and uterine microbiota from the same individuals were not as similar as expected [10]. Lately, the vaginal and endometrial microbiota of reproductive-age asymptomatic women have been compared to 16S rRNA sequencing of paired endometrial fluid and vaginal aspirates samples obtained under aseptic conditions [13]. Bacteria were detected in 100 per cent of the samples analysed, demonstrating once again that the endometrium is not sterile. As previously described, *Lactobacillus* was the most-represented genus in both endometrial and vaginal samples, followed by *Gardnerella, Atopobium, Clostridium* and *Prevotella*, among others, while *Propionibacterium, Acinetobacter* and some other genera were detected only in endometrial samples and not in their vaginal counterparts. Significant differences in the microbial profiles of paired endometrial and vaginal samples were observed, demonstrating that although closely related, the bacterial composition of the endometrium and vagina are not always identical [13].

Once the existence of an endometrial microbiome has been accepted, the role of these bacteria in the onset of several gynaecological and obstetrical diseases is beginning to be unravelled. An example of this can be found in the studies associating pathological shifts of endometrial microbiota and decreased abundance of *Lactobacilli*, with endometrial hyperplasia and endometrial cancer [14]. Also, the relevance of the human microbiome has been recognized all through the reproductive process, including gametes formation, fertilization, acquisition of endometrial receptivity, embryo implantation, pregnancy success and labour

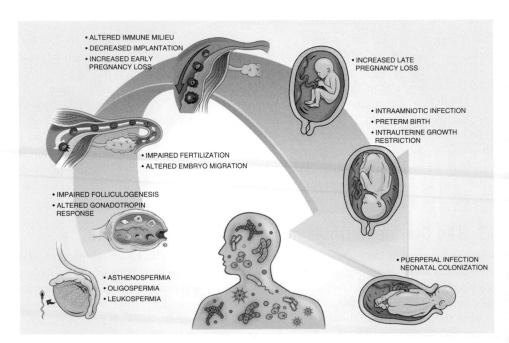

Figure 6.3 Diagram of the symbiotic relationship between host and bacteria in human reproduction
Source: Reprinted from Fertility and Sterility, 104(6), Franasiak JM, Scott RT Jr., Introduction: Microbiome in human reproduction, 1341–1343, Copyright 2015, with permission from Elsevier.

(Figure 6.3). The study of the reproductive tract microbiome, especially the uterine microbiome, will open new avenues in the near future to the improved management of infertile and pregnant patients.

6.3.1 Impact of the Uterine Microbiota in Pregnancy

The vaginal microbiome has been shown to be highly stable during pregnancy, reaching the minimum bacterial diversity represented by enriched *Lactobacillus* spp. from CST-I, -II, -III and -V in term pregnancies, while typical CST-IV polymicrobial communities have been associated with increased risk of early and late miscarriage and preterm birth (PTB; reviewed in [15]). Very few studies connecting the microbiome at the maternal-fetal interphase with pregnancy outcomes have been published to date, but their results have shown that the intrauterine microbiome has to be considered as a key factor in fertility, pregnancy maintenance and neonatal health.

6.3.1.1 Placental and Fetal Membranes Microbiota

Previous works have reported the existence of a low, but still active, microbiota surrounding the fetus not only in placental, membranes or amniotic fluid infections but also in normal pregnancies to term. Bacteria from Actinobacteria (*Bifidobacterium* spp.), Bacteroidetes (*Flavobacterium* spp.), Firmicutes (*Lactobacillus* spp.), Fusobacteria, Protcobacteria (*Escherichia* and *Neisseria* spp.) and Tenericutes (*Mycoplasma* spp.) phyla are the commensal bacteria colonizing the placenta in healthy pregnancies, while *Burkholderia, Roseovarius* and *Streptosporangium* are highly associated with preterm delivery [16]. Due to the similarity of the microbial profile found in the placenta with that in the oral cavity, it has been suggested that the placenta could be colonized by haematogenous spread at the time of vascularization during the formation of the placenta [16].

Also, colonization of the fetal membranes from ascending vaginal bacteria and colonizing the gravid intrauterine environment has been reported [17]. In this regard, chorioamnionitis is caused by polymicrobial growth of bacterial pathogens, i.e. *Streptococcus, Fusobacterium, Ureaplasma, Corynebacterium, E. coli, Peptostreptococcus, Prevotella* and genital *Mycoplasmas* [18], leading to inflammation of the chorion and amnion and premature rupture of membranes [19].

Pre-eclampsia is another example of obstetrical complication recently related to alterations in the microbiome. The bacterial taxa differentially found in pre-eclamptic patient are highly variable, including *Actinobacillus, Anoxybacillus, Bacillus, Dialister, Escherichia, Fusobacterium, Klebsiella, Listeria, Porphyromonas, Prevotella, Salmonella, Tannerella, Treponema* and *Variovorax* in the placenta, and *L. iners*, and bacteria from *Leptotrichia, Sneathia, Streptococcus* and *Ureaplasma* are more frequently detected in the amniotic fluid. The vast diversity of intrauterine bacteria found in pre-eclampsia hinders the association of specific taxa profiles to this disease, and, as a consequence, the existence of simultaneous dysbiotic agents has been postulated to cause the cellular events responsible for impaired endothelial function and increased blood pressure in gravid women [19, 20].

PTB constitutes one of the leading causes of morbidity and mortality of children younger than five years of age (World Health Organization, www.who.int). PTB has been linked to decreased intrauterine abundance of *L. crispatus* affecting choriodecidual space, amnion, chorion, placenta, amniotic fluid, umbilical cord, placenta or fetus, in favour of other infectious agents as *Bacteroides* spp., *E. coli, Fusobacterium nucleatum, G. vaginalis, Mycoplasma hominis, Sneathia sanguinegens, Streptococcus* spp., *Ureaplasma urealyticum* and *Ureaplasma parvum* [21, 12, 18]. The impact of bacterial infections in preterm labour could be triggered by the production of pro-inflammatory cytokines and prostaglandins that initiate uterine contractility and breakdown of the cervical epithelial barrier [19].

6.3.2 The Uterine Microbiota in Assisted Reproductive Techniques

The impact of the uterine microbiota in the aetiology of infertility has recently attracted a great focus of attention. Uterine infection has been traditionally proposed as a risk factor for impaired reproduction function, as this pathogenic environment may lead to the secretion of pro-inflammatory cytokines and the activation of the immune response in the uterus, thus altering embryo implantation and the onset of a successful pregnancy [22]. For that reason, the screening of the uterine microbiome as a part of the assisted reproductive techniques (ARTs) will improve the future clinical management of those patients whose infertility could have an origin in bacterial dysbiosis.

6.3.2.1 Chronic Endometritis

Chronic endometritis (CE) is produced by the microbial infection of the uterine lining by different kinds of yeast (Saccharomyces and Candida), common bacteria (*Enterococcus faecalis, Escherichia coli, Gardnerella vaginalis, Klebsiella pneumoniae, Proteus* spp., *Pseudomonas aeruginosa, Staphylococcus* spp. and *Streptococcus* spp.) and genital pathogens (*Neisseria gonorrhoeae, Chlamydia trachomatis* and *Ureaplasma urealyticum*). It has been reported that CE affects up to 45 per cent of infertile patients, but because this is usually asymptomatic and undetectable by ultrasound monitoring, this number could be even higher. Several mechanisms have been proposed as responsible for impaired reproduction function in CE patients, the most important being the dysregulation of proliferation, apoptosis and inflammation, mediated by the presence of pathogenic taxa in the endometrium. This is supported by the improvement of ART outcomes in those infertile patients with recurrent pregnancy loss (RPL) or repeated implantation failure (RIF) upon treatment with antibiogram-driven antibiotic therapy for CE [23].

6.3.2.2 Endometriosis

Endometriosis is a severe gynaecological condition in which endometrial tissues, epithelium and stroma are seeded and spread outside the uterine cavity forming cysts called endometriomas. This disease, affecting 10 per cent of reproductive-age women, is a direct cause of infertility [24]. Although the origin of endometriosis remains unknown, the latest knowledge on the uterine microbiome has proposed the presence of endometrial pathogens as one of the potential causes of endometriosis. This hypothesis is supported by the enriched detection of bacterial pathogens such as *E. coli, Gardnerella, Enterococcus, Streptococcus, Staphylococcus, Actinomyces, Corynebacterium, Fusobacterium, Prevotella* and *Propionibacterium*, together with decreased *Lactobacilli* in endometrial samples from endometriosis patients compared to a control group [25].

6.3.2.3 Endometrial Cavity Fluid

Endometrial cavity fluid (ECF) consists in the accumulation of secretion inside the uterine cavity coming from the fallopian tubes (hydrosalpinx), the ovaries, the cervix or even the endometrium. In some cases, ECF is originated by pelvic tuberculosis, chlamydia, gonorrhoea and other subclinical uterine infections. Despite ECF not being a common complication of ART patients, it has been shown to negatively impact implantation and pregnancy rates, and is responsible for increased early pregnancy loss. The poor reproductive outcomes of ECF patients could be explained by the embryotoxic effect of microorganisms, cytokines (IL-2, NF-κB and LIF) and endotoxins contained in this fluid. A concomitant effect is the mechanical factor complicating embryo adhesion due to the reduced presence of integrins in ECF patients, which in turn results in reduced endometrial receptivity [26, 23].

6.3.2.4 Repeated Implantation Failure and Recurrent Pregnancy Loss

Based on culture-dependent techniques, overt intrauterine infections have been traditionally associated with infertility and poor reproductive outcomes in in vitro fertilization (IVF) patients. In this regard, several studies consistently showed that isolation of Enterobacteriaceae, *Streptococcus* spp., *Staphylococcus* spp., *E. coli* and other anaerobic Gram-negative or Gram-positive bacteria from the embryo transfer catheter tip correlated with decreased implantation and pregnancy rates and increased miscarriage rates per transfer compared to negative cultures [15].

In the era of 16S rRNA gene metagenomics, the endometrial microbiome and its impact on ART success has been assessed in a bunch of studies. The endometrial microbiome of non-pregnant women with RIF and/or RPL has been described by target sequencing of the V1–V2 regions of the 16S rRNA genes, revealing that the uterine microbiome is mainly composed of bacteria from the Firmicutes, Bacteroidetes and Proteobacteria phyla [27].

The first study on the impact of the endometrial microbiome in ART was conducted by sequencing of the distal tip of the embryo catheter at the time of embryo transfer of IVF patients [28]. In this study, *Flavobacterium* and *Lactobacillus* were the most abundant taxa detected, followed by other typical genital tract bacteria. However, after applying multiple correction tests on the generated data, no differential bacterial profiles were associated with patients with ongoing versus non-ongoing pregnancies [28]. A second study sequencing of the V3–V5 hypervariable regions of the 16S rRNA gene on endometrial fluid samples collected in the receptive phase of IVF patients with RIF has enabled the classification of endometrial microbiome into *Lactobacillus* dominated (LD) and non-*Lactobacillus* dominated (NLD) based on their relative abundance of *Lactobacilli*, with a cut-off value of 90 per cent [13]. Following these criteria, patients were assigned an endometrial microbiota profile, and the reproductive outcome was compared between the LD and NLD group. The results of this study showed that patients whose IVF treatment resulted in live birth presented significantly increased levels of *Lactobacillus* spp. than those who did not become pregnant or suffer a miscarriage (Figure 6.4), which presented increased percentages of other dysbiotic bacteria as *Gardnerella* or *Streptococcus*. Interestingly, patients in the NLD endometrial microbiota group presented decreased implantation, pregnancy, ongoing pregnancy and live birth rates (23.1 vs. 60.7 per cent, $p = 0.02$; 33.3 vs. 70.6 per cent, $p = 0.03$; 13.3 vs. 58.8 per cent, $p = 0.02$; and 6.7 vs. 58.8 per cent, $p = 0.002$, respectively) than patients in the LD group [13]. Although further studies are needed for the validation of these data, the results of this study suggest that dysbiotic shifts of the normal uterine microbiome may induce

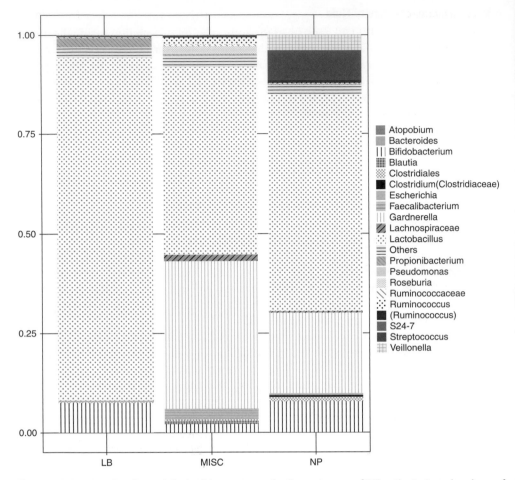

Figure 6.4 **Impact of endometrial microbiota on reproductive outcomes of IVF patients.** Low abundance of endometrial Lactobacillus is associated with poor reproductive outcome (LB: live birth, MISC: miscarriage; NP: non-pregnant)
Source: Reprinted from American Journal of Obstetrics & Gynecology, 215(6), Moreno I, Codoñer FM, Vilella F, et al., Evidence that the endometrial microbiota has an effect on implantation success or failure, 684–703, Copyright 2016, with permission from Elsevier.

molecular and/or cellular events impairing embryo implantation even in patients with a receptive endometrium.

6.4 Concluding Remarks

Recent advent of massive parallel sequencing, together with the knowledge of bacterial genomes, has facilitated the discovery of unique microbiomes in sterile-considered body niches, like the uterine microbiome. The study of the endometrial microbiome in IVF patients has revealed that bacterial communities may have an impact on reproductive success and failure, and, specifically, the presence of dysbiotic or pathogenic bacteria is now proposed as an emerging cause of repeated implantation failure or recurrent miscarriage. Taking into account the technical improvements on NGS technology and its increasing cost-effectiveness, the assessment of the uterine microbiome is foreseen as a growing field for the study of bacterial–host interactions in human reproduction and its clinical translation to improve the endometrial preparation of the endometrium for ART.

References

[1] Human Microbiome Project Consortium. Structure, function and diversity of the healthy human microbiome. *Nature* 2012; 486:207–14.

[2] Mor A, Driggers PH, Segars JH. Molecular characterization of the human microbiome from a reproductive perspective. *Fertil Steril* 2015;104:1344–50.

[3] Franasiak JM, Scott RT Jr. Introduction: Microbiome in human reproduction. *Fertil Steril* 2015;104:1341–3.

[4] Sirota I, Zarek SM, Segars JH. Potential influence of the microbiome on infertility and assisted reproductive technology. *Semin Reprod Med* 2014;32:35–42.

[5] Miles SM, Hardy BL, Merrell DS. Investigation of the microbiota of the reproductive tract in women undergoing a total hysterectomy and bilateral salpingo-oopherectomy. *Fertil Steril* 2017;107:813–20.

[6] Ravel J, Gajer P, Abdo Z et al. Vaginal microbiome of reproductive-age women. *Proc Natl Acad Sci USA* 2011;108:4680–7.

[7] Gajer P, Brotman RM, Bai G et al. Temporal dynamics of the human vaginal microbiota. *Sci Transl Med* 2012;4:132ra52.

[8] Romero R, Hassan SS, Gajer P et al. The composition and stability of the vaginal microbiota of normal pregnant women is different from that of non-pregnant women. *Microbiome* 2014;2:4.

[9] Green KA, Zarek SM, Catherino WH. Gynecologic health and disease in relation to the microbiome of the female reproductive tract. *Fertil Steril* 2015;104:1351–7.

[10] Mitchell CM, Haick A, Nkwopara E et al. Colonization of the upper genital tract by vaginal bacterial species in nonpregnant women. *Am J Obstet Gynecol* 2015;212:611.e1–9.

[11] Pelzer ES, Allan JA, Cunningham K et al. Microbial colonization of follicular fluid: alterations in cytokine expression and adverse assisted reproduction technology outcomes. *Hum Reprod* 2011;26:1799–812.

[12] Swidsinski A, Verstraelen H, Loening-Baucke V et al. Presence of a polymicrobial endometrial biofilm in patients with bacterial vaginosis. *PLoS One* 2013;8:e53997.

[13] Moreno I, Codoñer FM, Vilella F et al. Evidence that the endometrial microbiota has an effect on implantation success or failure. *Am J Obstet Gynecol* 2016;215:684–703.

[14] Walther-António MRS, Chen J, Multinu F et al. Potential contribution of the uterine microbiome in the development of endometrial cancer. *Genome Med* 2016;8:122.

[15] Moreno I, Simon C, Microbiological diagnosis: The human endometrial microbiome–Endometritis, in Simon C, Giudice LC, eds, *The Endometrial Factor: A Reproductive Precision Medicine Approach*, CRC Press: Boca Raton, 2017: 65–77.

[16] Aagaard K, Ma J, Antony KM et al. The placenta harbors a unique microbiome. *Sci Transl Med* 2014;6:237ra65.

[17] Solt I. The human microbiome and the great obstetrical syndromes: a new frontier in maternal-fetal medicine. *Best Pract Res Clin Obstet Gynaecol* 2015;29:165–75.

[18] Prince AL, Ma J, Kannan PS et al. The placental membrane microbiome is altered among subjects with spontaneous preterm birth with and without chorioamnionitis. *Am J Obstet Gynecol* 2016;214:627.e1–627.

[19] Moreno I, Franasiak JM. The endometrial microbiota – New player in town. *Fertil Steril* 2017; in press.

[20] Amarasekara R, Jayasekara RW et al. Microbiome of the placenta in pre-eclampsia supports the role of bacteria in the multifactorial cause of pre-eclampsia. *J Obstet Gynaecol Res* 2015;41:662–9.

[21] Goldenberg RL, Culhane JF, Iams JD, Romero R. Epidemiology and causes of preterm birth. *Lancet* 2008;371:75–84.

[22] Franasiak JM, Scott RT Jr. Reproductive tract microbiome in assisted reproductive technologies. *Fertil Steril* 2015;104:1364–71.

[23] Akopians AL, Pisarska MD, Wang ET. The Role of Inflammatory Pathways in Implantation Failure: Chronic Endometritis and Hydrosalpinges. *Semin Reprod Med* 2015;33:298–304.

[24] Fuldeore MJ, Soliman AM. Prevalence and Symptomatic Burden of Diagnosed Endometriosis in the United States: National Estimates from a Cross-Sectional Survey of 59,411 Women. Gynecologic and Obstetric Investigation 2016.

[25] Khan KN, Fujishita A, Masumoto H et al. Molecular detection of intrauterine microbial colonization in women with endometriosis. *Eur J Obstet Gynecol Reprod Biol* 2016;199:69–75.

[26] Liu S, Shi L, Shi J. Impact of endometrial cavity fluid on assisted reproductive technology outcomes. *Int J Gynecol Obstet* 2016;132:278–83.

[27] Verstraelen H, Vilchez-Vargas R, Desimpel F et al. Characterisation of the human uterine microbiome in non-pregnant women through deep sequencing of the V1-2 region of the 16S rRNA gene. *PeerJ* 2016;4:e1602.

[28] Franasiak JM, Werner MD, Juneau CR et al. Endometrial microbiome at the time of embryo transfer: Next-generation sequencing of the 16S ribosomal subunit. *J Assist Reprod Genet* 2016;33:129–36.

Chapter

7

Estrogen and Progesterone Support in ART
Optimizing Implantation

Jamie Stanhiser and Steven L. Young

7.1 Introduction

The endometrium undergoes dynamic structural and functional changes throughout the menstrual cycle, directed primarily by the ovarian steroid hormones, estradiol (E_2) and progesterone (P_4), as illustrated in Figure 7.1. Estrogen is the primary regulator of proliferative-phase endometrium, inducing stromal and epithelial proliferation, endometrial neoangiogenesis, and preparing the endometrium for the secretory phase by inducing expression of P_4 receptors. Following ovulation, P_4 in addition to estrogen is secreted by the corpus luteum, resulting in induction of secretory vacuole formation, a halting of epithelial proliferation, alterations in resident immune cell composition, increased stromal

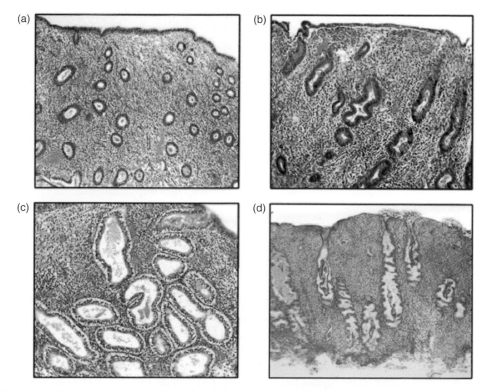

Figure 7.1 Light micrographs of endometrium at the following cycle stages
A. Early proliferative; B. Late proliferative; C. Early secretory; D. Late secretory

edema, and dense coiling of the spiral arteries. These secretory phase changes result in a two- to three-day period of optimal endometrial receptivity for embryo implantation that is temporally synchronized with blastocyst readiness. In contrast to the highly synchronized development of the endometrium and embryo in a natural cycle, controlled ovarian stimulation (COS) during assisted reproductive technology (ART) cycles exposes the endometrium to a markedly altered hormonal milieu, with the potential to change both the qualitative and the temporal aspects of endometrial receptivity. The development of many follicles results in an endometrium exposed to markedly higher E_2 than that seen in natural cycles, while premature luteinization can cause a temporal shift in the endometrial exposure to P_4. Gonadotropin-releasing hormone analogues (GnRHa) used in ART, combined with removal of granulosa cells during oocyte retrieval, can result in an earlier decline in E_2 and P_4 production by the corpus luteum, further altering the endometrial environment [1,2]. Taken together, these alterations in hormonal milieu can result in significant changes in endometrial receptivity. Understanding the altered physiology associated with ART provides a basis for improved embryo implantation and optimization of clinical outcomes.

7.2 Progesterone in IVF

The confluence of evidence from epidemiology and study of oocyte donation and frozen embryo transfer cycles demonstrate that continued luteal phase P_4 exposure results in a two- to three-day temporal window of normal uterine receptivity. Further, synchrony between endometrial and embryo readiness is critical to the establishment of pregnancy [3]. Therefore, many have hypothesized that a premature elevation of P_4 levels prior to ovulation trigger, seen in some ART cycles, might alter endometrial-embryo synchrony by temporally advancing the endometrial receptivity window. Three theories have been proposed to explain follicular-phase P_4 elevation during ART stimulation (premature luteinization) despite GnRH analog suppression of LH secretion: increased sensitivity of granulosa cell LH receptor to follicle-stimulating hormone (FSH); the accumulation of human chorionic gonadotrophin (hCG) in the serum from human menopausal gonadotropin (hMG) administration; and decreased conversion of P_4 to androgens in theca cells due to GnRHa suppression of LH. Interestingly, the type of gonadotropin may affect the rate of premature luteinization, as higher serum P_4 is observed in patients treated with recombinant FSH rather than highly purified (HP)-hMG in both GnRH agonist and antagonist cycles [4], although these observational data may be biased by the types of patients that are clinically selected for each protocol.

Studies examining the impact of early P_4 production have demonstrated discrepant findings, likely due to different cutoff criteria used to define "elevated" P_4, and different assay methodology. Many early studies found a statistically nonsignificant trend toward lower pregnancy rates with elevated P_4. More recently, studies have identified a significantly lower ART pregnancy rate in patients with elevated serum P_4 concentrations. In a retrospective analysis of over 4000 ART patients, Bosch and colleagues demonstrated a strong, dose-dependent association between serum P_4 greater than 1.5 ng/mL on the day of hCG administration and lower pregnancy rates (Figure 7.2) [5]. Elevated levels of P_4 were found to be associated with the use of GnRH agonist (rather than antagonist) as well as higher serum E_2 concentration, FSH dose, and number of oocytes retrieved [5]. A 2013 meta-analysis of over 60,000 cycles found that P_4 elevation on the day of hCG administration is associated with a decreased probability of pregnancy in fresh in vitro fertilization

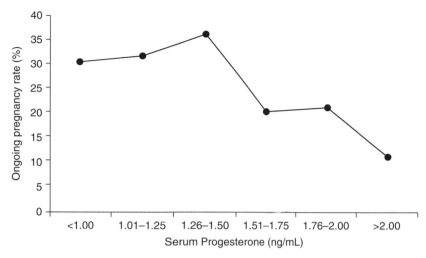

Figure 7.2 Serum P_4 on day of hCG administration and ongoing pregnancy rates
Source: Data from Bosch et al.

(IVF) cycles; however, the pregnancy rates from subsequent transfer of frozen-thawed embryos originating from that cycle were not affected [6]. These results suggest that elevated P_4 levels have an adverse affect on the maternal endometrium rather than the oocyte. The lack of effect on oocyte quality was further supported by comparing paired oocyte recipient outcomes from donors who demonstrated elevated P_4 in one cycle, but not the other [7]. The cited studies strongly support the concept that premature elevation of P_4 reduces ART success, and we recommend use of serum P_4 measurement on the day of trigger to optimize clinical decisions between fresh transfer and cryopreservation of all embryos. Although different cutoff levels have been proposed, we have found excellent results by converting to a frozen transfer cycle with P_4 serum concentrations > 1.5 ng/mL.

Following the administration of hCG for induction of final oocyte maturation, P_4 levels rise rapidly. However, use of GnRHa may shorten the luteal phase, with GnRH antagonist posing a greater risk than agonist [2]. It has also been hypothesized that removal of granulosa cells during oocyte retrieval may further compromise corpora luteal function [1]. A systematic review demonstrated significantly improved clinical pregnancy and live birth rates with luteal phase P_4 support [8]. Because of this, luteal phase P_4 support is routine, with P_4 supplementation administered by various routes and at multiple doses [1,9].

Optimal timing of P_4 supplementation initiation during ART has been studied, and it begins on the evening after oocyte retrieval and ends by the third day after retrieval [10,11]. However, the optimal length of time for P_4 support of pregnancy after ART is not clearly delineated. Kohls and colleagues compared stopping luteal phase P_4 support at five weeks versus eight weeks after oocyte retrieval, and there was no difference in ongoing pregnancy rates between groups; however, there was significantly more bleeding in the five-week group [12]. Because first-trimester bleeding commonly induces anxiety in both the patient and clinician, P_4 supplementation beyond five weeks after retrieval is widely used.

Historically, P_4 was given using daily intramuscular injections of 50–100 mg in oil over several weeks. However, injections are associated with patient discomfort, and alternative modes of P_4 administration have been evaluated. Oral P_4 supplementation is associated with reduced implantation rates [13], consistent with known pharmacokinetic and metabolic variability. Randomized trial of IVF outcomes demonstrated that P_4 supplementation via a "bioadhesive" vaginal gel preparation (Crinone®) appears equivalent to intramuscular injection [9, 14]. Similarly, a meta-analysis comparing routes of P_4 supplementation administration found no difference in pregnancy rates between vaginal preparations and intramuscular injection, or between different vaginal micronized P_4 suppositories [15]. While vaginal administration appears equivalent to intramuscular in IVF, outcomes in frozen embryo or donor oocyte cycles are less clear, with a possible benefit of intramuscular preparations [9, 16].

7.3 Estrogen in IVF

The multiple follicular development resulting from COS in ART commonly causes serum E_2 concentrations to exceed that seen in natural cycles by five– tenfold. Very high follicular-phase estrogen concentrations are associated with poorer pregnancy rates, though the mechanism remains unknown and results differ between centers [17]. Effects of altered luteal phase E_2 in IVF cycles are also controversial. The same factors that reduce and/or shorten corpus luteum production of P_4 have the same effect on E_2 production. A prospective randomized study of GnRHa IVF cycles compared luteal-phase E_2 supplementation of 0, 2, and 6 mg and found that pregnancy rates were improved by E_2 supplementation in a dose-related fashion, with the highest pregnancy rates in the 6 mg estrogen supplement group [18]. Another randomized trial in GnRH agonist IVF cycles found that adjunctive supplementation with E_2 in the luteal phase resulted in higher implantation and pregnancy rates with lower miscarriage rate than P_4 supplementation alone [19]. However, more recent randomized clinical trials and meta-analyses have found no benefit [20,21]. Thus, it remains unclear if luteal E_2 supplementation has any benefit in fresh IVF cycles and we do not use it in our clinic.

7.4 Estrogen and Progesterone Supplementation in Frozen-Thawed, Donor-Recipient, and Gestational Carrier Cycles

In fresh embryo transfer cycles, the corpora lutea are a rich source of endogenous estrogen and progesterone; however, in frozen, donor, or gestational carrier cycles there is typically no corpus luteum and endogenous ovarian hormone production is prevented by GnRHa use and/or suppressed by the exogenous estrogen and progesterone support. Therefore, estrogen and progesterone dosing and timing in frozen, donor, and gestational carrier cycles are different than in fresh cycles, to ensure synchronization of embryo development with endometrial receptivity for implantation. Preparing the endometrium with a standard E_2 and P_4 regimen results in endometrial exposure to steroid concentrations more closely resembling a natural cycle, and, in one recent randomized controlled trial, pregnancy rates following primary frozen embryo transfer were significantly higher (84 percent) than those with primary fresh embryo transfer (55 percent) [22]. The transfer of cryopreserved embryos may also be performed in a natural menstrual cycle. A recent systematic review found no difference between natural menstrual cycle and various controlled regimens [22], though there are clear scheduling benefits for the patient and clinic using exogenous steroid hormone therapies. For both oocyte donor-recipient and gestational carrier cycles, the need to control the timing of receptivity of the recipient uterus requires a controlled E_2 and P_4 supplement regimen, unless frozen oocytes or embryos are used and replaced in an ovulatory natural cycle.

7.5 Assessing Alterations in the Window of Implantation

The window of implantation (WOI) is the discreet time period during which the receptivity of the endometrium is synchronized with embryo development to enable embryo implantation. Identification of this window of endometrial receptivity offers many challenges, and most proposed methods of diagnosis are limited by their invasive nature, lack of accuracy, and poor predictive value. Noyes, Hertig, and Rock first established histologic criteria to evaluate endometrial development and receptivity [23]. However, the precision of these histologic markers was critically reanalyzed, challenged, and largely invalidated [24,25; Figure 7.3]. Ultrasound characteristics associated with endometrial receptivity such as endometrial thickness and blood flow patterns have been identified; however, they have not clearly demonstrated clinical value.

The duration of P_4 exposure is clearly the main determinant of the timing of the WOI. Some of the most persuasive data include examination of the success of embryo transfer in oocyte donation cycles. Prappas et al. demonstrated a two-day peak (Figure 7.4) receptivity to embryo implantation, mirroring findings in natural cycles regarding day of implantation [26,27].

Recently, microarray technology has enabled the development of a molecular diagnostic test to evaluate the endometrium and specifically identify the WOI, called the endometrial receptivity array (ERA), which has been found to be superior to previous methodologies [28,

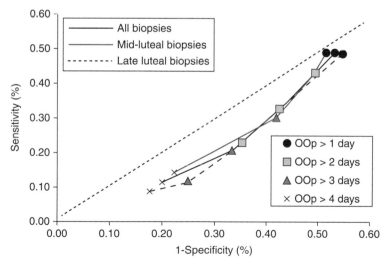

Figure 7.3 Histological dating of endometrial biopsy tissue showing poor sensitivity and specificity for classifying infertility by a biopsy out of phase (OOP) by more than one to four days. The dotted diagonal line represents a test that does not discriminate between true and false positives
Source: Reprinted with Permission, Coutifaris et al.

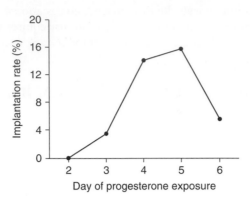

Figure 7.4 Duration of progesterone exposure and implantation rate
Source: Data from Prappas et al.

29]. ERA has been used in studies to evaluate endometrial receptivity in natural cycles compared with IVF cycles, and have identified that IVF cycles have altered transcriptional activity of genes involved with endometrial receptivity, and may be altered in different types of COS protocols [30]. Using ERA in patients with recurrent implantation failure, the WOI was found to be significantly displaced in a quarter of patients, and the use of an adjusted personalized embryo transfer on the day designated by ERA improved reproductive outcomes [31]. Studies on the accuracy of ERA are promising; however, randomized controlled trials are necessary prior to its wide application in the clinical setting. This is discussed in Chapter 4.

Other factors, independent of shifting the implantation window, may impact endometrial receptivity and fecundability. Intrauterine adhesive disease has been found to alter the surrounding endometrium, and women with this disease often have difficulty proliferating their endometrium despite long courses of estrogen. Endometrial thickness measurements of less than 6.5–7 mm are associated with decreased pregnancy rates; it has been proposed that exposure of the basal layer of endometrium might lead to higher levels of reactive oxygen species [32]. Replenishing endometrium with stem cells is an exciting new possibility in the early stages of development [33]. Other factors, independent of injury or sex steroids may alter endometrial receptivity. The presence of endometriosis lesions, associated with regional and systemic inflammation, seems to be associated with altered endometrial response to P_4 and reduced efficiency of implantation, though much work needs to be done to understand the impact of these findings and whether altered P_4 supplementation might be beneficial [34].

7.6 Conclusion

Translating our knowledge about the roles of estrogen and P_4 in receptivity to embryo implantation has allowed significant progress in the optimization of infertility and subfertility treatment. Despite this optimization, recent studies suggest that more than a third of euploid embryos fail to implant properly, for reasons that remain unclear. Thus, there is substantial clinical opportunity in gaining further detail about the role of estrogen, P_4, and other factors in the determination of endometrial receptivity.

References

1. Van Steirteghem AC, Smitz J, Camus M et al. The luteal phase after in-vitro fertilization and related procedures. *Hum Reprod* 1988;3:161–164.

2. Beckers NGM, Macklon NS, Eijkemans MJ et al. Nonsupplemented luteal phase characteristics after the administration of recombinant human chorionic gonadotropin, recombinant luteinizing hormone, or gonadotropin-releasing hormone (GnRH) agonist to induce final oocyte maturation in in vitro fertilization patients after ovarian stimulation with recombinant follicle stimulating hormone and GnRH antagonist cotreatment. *Journal of Clinical Endocrinology and Metabolism* 2003;88:4186–4192.

3. Bergh PA, Navot D. The impact of embryonic development and endometrial maturity on the timing of implantation. *Fertil Steril* 1992;58:537–542.

4. Andersen AN, Devroey P, Arce JC. Clinical outcome following stimulation with highly purified hMG or recombinant FSH in patients undergoing IVF: a randomized assessor-blind controlled trial. *Hum Reprod* 2006;21:3217–3227.

5. Bosch E, Labarta E, Crespo J et al. Circulating progesterone levels and ongoing pregnancy rates in controlled ovarian stimulation cycles for in vitro fertilization: analysis of over 4000 cycles. *Hum Reprod* 2010;25:2092–2100.

6. Venetis CA, Kolibianakis EM, Bosdou JK, Tarlatzis BC. Progesterone elevation and probability of pregnancy after IVF: a systematic review and meta-analysis of over 60 000 cycles. *Hum Reprod Update* 2013;19:433–457.

7. Melo MA, Meseguer M, Garrido N et al. The significance of premature luteinization in an oocyte-donation programme. *Hum Reprod* 2006;21:1503–1507.

8. van der Linden M, Buckingham K, Farquhar C, Kremer JA, Metwally M. Luteal phase support for assisted reproduction cycles. *Cochrane Database Syst Rev* 2011 October 5;(10):CD009154.doi(10): CD009154.

9. Yanushpolsky E, Hurwitz S, Greenberg L, Racowsky C, Hornstein M. Crinone vaginal gel is equally effective and better tolerated than intramuscular progesterone for luteal phase support in in vitro fertilization-embryo transfer cycles: a prospective randomized study. *Fertil Steril* 2010;94:2596–2599.

10. Sohn SH, Penzias AS, Emmi AM et al. Administration of progesterone before oocyte retrieval negatively affects the implantation rate. *Fertil Steril* 1999;71:11–14.

11. Williams SC, Oehninger S, Gibbons WE, Van Cleave WC, Muasher SJ. Delaying the initiation of progesterone supplementation results in decreased pregnancy rates after in vitro fertilization: a randomized, prospective study. *Fertil Steril* 2001;76:1140–1143.

12. Kohls G, Ruiz F, Martinez M et al. Early progesterone cessation after in vitro fertilization/intracytoplasmic sperm injection: a randomized, controlled trial. *Fertil Steril* 2012;98:858–862.

13. Licciardi FL, Kwiatkowski A, Noyes NL et al. Oral versus intramuscular progesterone for in vitro fertilization: a prospective randomized study. *Fertil Steril* 1999;71:614–618.

14. Kahraman S, Karagozoglu SH, Karlikaya G. The efficiency of progesterone vaginal gel versus intramuscular progesterone for luteal phase supplementation in gonadotropin-releasing hormone antagonist cycles: a prospective clinical trial. *Fertil Steril.* 2010;94:761–763.

15. Zarutskie PW, Phillips JA. A meta-analysis of the route of administration of luteal phase support in assisted reproductive technology: vaginal versus intramuscular progesterone. *Fertil Steril* 2009;92:163–169.

16. Casper RF, Yanushpolsky EH. Optimal endometrial preparation for frozen embryo transfer cycles: window of implantation and progesterone support. *Fertil Steril.* 2016;105:867–872.

17. Simón C, Cano F, Valbuena D, Remohí J, Pellicer A. Clinical evidence for a detrimental effect on uterine receptivity

of high serum oestradiol concentrations in high and normal responder patients. *Hum Reprod.* 1995;10:2432–2437.

18. Lukaszuk K, Liss J, Lukaszuk M, Maj B. Optimization of estradiol supplementation during the luteal phase improves the pregnancy rate in women undergoing in vitro fertilization–embryo transfer cycles. *Fertil Steril* 2005;83:1372–1376.

19. Ghanem ME, Sadek EE, Elboghdady LA et al. The effect of luteal phase support protocol on cycle outcome and luteal phase hormone profile in long agonist protocol intracytoplasmic sperm injection cycles: a randomized clinical trial. *Fertil Steril* 2009;92:486–493.

20. Tonguc E, Var T, Ozyer S, Citil A, Dogan M. Estradiol supplementation during the luteal phase of in vitro fertilization cycles: a prospective randomised study. *European Journal of Obstetrics & Gynecology and Reproductive Biology* 2011;154:172–176.

21. Gelbaya TA, Kyrgiou M, Tsoumpou I, Nardo LG. The use of estradiol for luteal phase support in in vitro fertilization/ intracytoplasmic sperm injection cycles: a systematic review and meta-analysis. *Fertil Steril* 2008;90:2116–2125.

22. Ghobara T, Vandekerckhove P. Cycle regimens for frozen-thawed embryo transfer. *Cochrane Database Syst Rev* 2008 January 23; (1):CD003414.doi(1): CD003414.

23. Noyes RW, Hertig AT, Rock J. Dating the endometrial biopsy. *Fertil Steril* 1950;1:3–25.

24. Murray MJ, Meyer WR, Zaino RJ et al. A critical analysis of the accuracy, reproducibility, and clinical utility of histologic endometrial dating in fertile women. *Fertil Steril.* 2004;81:1333–1343.

25. Coutifaris C, Myers ER, Guzick DS et al. Histological dating of timed endometrial biopsy tissue is not related to fertility status. *Fertil Steril* 2004;82:1264–1272.

26. Prappas N, Jones EE, Duleba AJ et al. Window for embryo transfer in oocyte donation cycles depends on the duration of progesterone therapy. *Hum Reprod.* 1998;13:720–723.

27. Wilcox AJ, Baird DD, Weinberg CR. Time of implantation of the conceptus and loss of pregnancy. *N Engl J Med.* 1999;340:1796–1799.

28. Díaz-Gimeno P, Ruiz-Alonso M, Blesa D et al. The accuracy and reproducibility of the endometrial receptivity array is superior to histology as a diagnostic method for endometrial receptivity. *Fertil Steril* 2013;99:508–517.

29. Evans GE, Martínez-Conejero JA, Phillipson GTM et al. Gene and protein expression signature of endometrial glandular and stromal compartments during the window of implantation. *Fertil Steril* 2012;97:1365–1373.e2.

30. Haouzi D, Assou S, Mahmoud K et al. Gene expression profile of human endometrial receptivity: comparison between natural and stimulated cycles for the same patients. *Hum Reprod* 2009;24:1436–1445.

31. Mahajan N. Endometrial receptivity array: Clinical application. *J Hum Reprod Sci* 2015;8:121–129.

32. Evans-Hoeker EA, Young SL. Endometrial receptivity and intrauterine adhesive disease. *Semin Reprod Med* 2014; 32:392–401.

33. Nagori CB, Panchal SY, Patel H. Endometrial regeneration using autologous adult stem cells followed by conception by in vitro fertilization in a patient with severe Asherman's syndrome. *J Hum Reprod Sci* 2011;4:43–48.

34. Fox C, Morin S, Jeong JW, Scott RT Jr, Lessey BA. Local and systemic factors and implantation: what is the evidence? *Fertil Steril.* 2016;105:873–884.

Chapter 8

The Role of Hysteroscopy and Endometrial Scratch in Improving Endometrial Receptivity

Yuval Or and Zeev Shoham

Evaluating the uterine cavity is a basic step when investigating all subfertile women, since the uterine cavity and the endometrium are both very important for the implantation of the human blastocyst [1].

Since the beginning of IVF, great improvements have been made in ovarian stimulation protocols and fertilization procedures. Despite such improvements, implantation remains the rate-limiting step for successful IVF treatments. Implantation is classified into three stages: apposition, adhesion and penetration. The uterus plays a critical role towards the success of each stage. To ensure that the endometrium will be receptive for blastocyst implantation, the endometrium must be initially stimulated by the ovarian steroids, oestrogen (E) and progesterone (P). These hormones induce the differentiation of endometrial stroma cells to form the decidua that provides the anatomical site for blastocyst implantation.

Implantation failure is generally related to inadequate endometrial receptivity in two-thirds of cases and abnormalities of the embryo in one-third [1]. A receptive endometrium is morphologically and functionally primed for blastocyst attachment. Many factors can affect the uterine cavity and the endometrial receptivity such as inappropriate hormonal stimulation, congenital uterine septum, submucosal fibroids, intrauterine adhesions and endometrial polyps. All these factors can negatively influence the embryo's ability to implant.

In this chapter, we will review the literature regarding the role of hysteroscopy and endometrial scratch in improving endometrial receptivity and IVF success rates.

8.1 The Role of Hysteroscopy in Improving Endometrial Receptivity

Hysteroscopy is performed to evaluate and treat the uterine cavity, tubal ostia and endocervical canal. It allows the direct visualization of the uterine cavity through a rigid, semi-rigid or flexible endoscope. Most diagnostic and many operative procedures can be done in an office setting using local anaesthesia and fluid distension media, while more complex procedures are generally performed as day surgeries under general anaesthesia [2]. Operative hysteroscopic procedures require a complex instrumentation set-up, special surgical training and appropriate knowledge and management of complications [3].

Hysteroscopy is the gold standard method for both diagnosis and treatment of intrauterine pathologies that may adversely affect fertility. Traditionally, hysteroscopy was reserved for treating diseases identified by other less invasive methods such as hysterosalpingography, transvaginal ultrasonography or saline sonohysterography. However, modern operative hysteroscopes, with an outer diameter measuring 2–3 mm, permit the safe performance of diagnostic and minor operative procedures [4].

It is assumed that major uterine cavity abnormalities may interfere with factors that regulate the blastocyst–endometrium communication. Many hypotheses have been formulated on how endometrial polyps, submucous fibroids, intrauterine adhesions and uterine septum are likely to disturb human embryo implantation. Nevertheless, the precise mechanisms of action through which each one of these major uterine cavity abnormalities affect this essential reproductive process are poorly understood [1].

When discussing whether women should be offered a routine hysteroscopy, we must consider the procedure's complications. Although complications from hysteroscopy are rare, they can potentially be life threatening. A multicentre study, including 13,600 diagnostic and operative hysteroscopic procedures performed in 82 centres, reported a complication rate of 0.28 per cent. Diagnostic hysteroscopy had a significantly lower complication rate compared to operative hysteroscopy (0.13 per cent vs. 0.95 per cent). The most common complication of both types of hysteroscopy was uterine perforation. Fluid intravasation occurred almost exclusively in operative procedures. Intrauterine adhesiolysis was associated with the highest incidence of complications while all other procedures had complication rates of less than 1 per cent [5,6].

8.2 Elective Hysteroscopy in a Normal Ultrasound Uterine Cavity

The British National Institute for Health and Clinical Excellence (NICE) guidelines on fertility assessment and treatment stated in 2004 that 'women should not be offered hysteroscopy on its own as part of the initial investigation of infertility unless clinically indicated because the effectiveness of surgical treatment of uterine abnormalities on improving pregnancy rates has not been established' [7].

In order to assess whether a routine hysteroscopy should be offered as part of an initial infertility investigation, Janine G Smith and colleagues performed a pragmatic, multicentre, randomized controlled trial. They compared 373 women who underwent hysteroscopy to 377 women who underwent immediate IVF. They found that 57 per cent of the 369 women eligible for assessment in the hysteroscopy group and 54 per cent of the immediate IVF group had a live birth from pregnancies during the trial period (relative risk 1·06, 95 per cent CI 0·93–1·20; $p=0·41$). One (<1 per cent) woman in the hysteroscopy group developed endometritis after hysteroscopy. They concluded that routine hysteroscopy does not improve live birth rates in infertile women with a normal transvaginal ultrasound of the uterine cavity scheduled for a first IVF treatment, and therefore women should not be offered routine hysteroscopies [8].

In order to determine whether hysteroscopies should be offered to women with recurrent implantation failure, Tarek El-Toukhy and colleagues performed a multicentre, randomized controlled trial. They recruited 702 women who had a normal ultrasound of the uterine cavity and a history of 2 to 4 unsuccessful IVF cycles. They then compared 350 women who received an outpatient hysteroscopy in the month before starting an IVF treatment cycle to 352 women in the control group who did not. Twenty-nine per cent of the women in the hysteroscopy group had a live birth after IVF compared with 29 per cent women in the control group (risk ratio 1·0, 95 per cent CI 0·79–1·25; p=0·96). No hysteroscopy-related adverse events were reported. They concluded that outpatient hysteroscopy before IVF in women with a normal ultrasound of the uterine cavity and a history of unsuccessful IVF treatment cycles does not improve the live birth rate [9].

8.3 Hysteroscopy in Major Uterine Cavity Abnormalities or Malformations

Major uterine cavity abnormalities can be found in 10–15 per cent of women seeking treatment for subfertility. Ultrasonography (US), preferably transvaginally (TVS), is used to screen for possible endometrium or uterine cavity abnormalities in the work-up of subfertile women. This evaluation can be expanded with hysterosalpingography (HSG), or saline infusion/gel instillation sonography (SIS/GIS). The NICE guidelines on fertility assessment and treatment stated in 2004 that there is a change towards diagnosis and treatment of all major uterine cavity abnormalities prior to fertility treatment. For endometrial polyps, submucous fibroids, intrauterine adhesions and uterine septum, observational studies have shown a clear improvement in the spontaneous pregnancy rate after the hysteroscopic removal of the abnormality [1].

8.4 Hysteroscopy in Endometrial Polyps

Endometrial polyps are the most common acquired uterine cavity abnormality. This benign, endometrial stalk-like mass protrudes into the uterine cavity and has its own vascular supply. Depending on the population under study and the applied diagnostic test, endometrial polyps can be found in 1–41 per cent of the subfertile population [10].

The Cochrane review in its systematic review – 'Hysteroscopy for treating subfertility associated with suspected major uterine cavity abnormalities', from 2015 [6] – found only one study that met the inclusion criteria regarding the hysteroscopic removal of polyps prior to intrauterine insemination (IUI) by Triso Perez-Medina and colleagues [11].

This study compared, in a prospective randomized trial, 101 patients who underwent hysteroscopic polypectomy to 103 patients who underwent diagnostic hysteroscopy and a polyp biopsy. They found that women had a better chance of becoming pregnant after polypectomy, with a relative risk of 2.1 (95 per cent confidence interval 1.5–2.9). About 29 per cent of women in the polypectomy group compared to 3 per cent in the diagnostic hysteroscopy group became pregnant in the three-month period after the hysteroscopy before starting treatment with gonadotropin and IUI, and the rest were obtained over a four-cycle period, without a clear distribution between the cycles. They concluded that 'pregnancies after polypectomy are frequently obtained spontaneously while waiting for the treatment, suggesting a strong cause–effect of the polyp in the implantation process and that hysteroscopic polypectomy before IUI is an effective measure' [11]. The Cochrane review in its systematic review concluded that there is a benefit for subfertile women with a sonographic diagnosis of endometrial polyps to undergo a hysteroscopic polypectomy to improve the chances of conceiving prior to intrauterine insemination for unexplained male or female factor infertility for at least 24 months [6].

8.5 Hysteroscopy in Submucosal Fibroids

Uterine fibroids are one of the most common benign tumours of the female genital tract, occurring in 20–50 per cent of women of reproductive age. Several theories have been proposed to explain how uterine fibroids may cause infertility, including deforming the uterine cavity, causing a hyperoestrogenic environment which may be responsible for the anovulatory cycles, pathological changes of the endometrium and myometrium such as atrophy of the endometrium, elongation and distortion of the glands, cystic glandular hyperplasia, polyposis, endometrial venule ectasia and ulceration and dysfunctional uterine contractility that may interfere with sperm migration, ovum transport or nidation. The anatomical location of the fibroid is an important factor in causing infertility in the following descending order: submucosal, intramural and subserosal. Submucosal fibroids may cause infertility for other reasons such as local inflammations caused by mucus ulceration altering the biochemical characteristics of intrauterine fluids, creating a hostile environment for the spermatozoa, and disruption of the endometrial blood supply, thereby affecting nidation of the embryo [12].

The Cochrane review in its systematic review – 'Hysteroscopy for treating subfertility associated with suspected major uterine cavity abnormalities', from 2015 – found only one study that met the inclusion criteria: women with otherwise unexplained subfertility and submucous fibroids by Casini et al. [6, 13].

The authors of this study performed a prospective controlled study to evaluate whether the location of uterine fibroids influences reproductive functions in women and whether removal of the fibroid prior to conception may improve the pregnancy rate and pregnancy maintenance. The patients in the intervention group were treated with hysteroscopic surgery to remove the fibroids and were encouraged to abstain from having sexual intercourse for three months and then start having regular fertility-oriented intercourse. Women in the control group were asked to immediately start having regular fertility-oriented intercourse. Both groups were monitored for up to 12 months. They recruited 181 patients with fibroids in various locations. Ninety-two patients underwent surgical treatment and 89 patients were not subject to surgical treatment. The pregnancy rates obtained were 43.3 per cent in cases of submucosal fibroids in patients who underwent myomectomy versus 27.2 per cent in patients who did not undergo surgical treatment ($p<0.05$); in cases of intramural fibroids, 56.5 per cent versus 41.0 per cent (NS); in cases of submucosal–intramural, 40.0 per cent versus 15.0 per cent ($p<0.05$); and in cases of intramural–subserosal uterine fibroids, 35.5 per cent versus 21.43 per cent (NS), respectively. The study authors concluded that the pregnancy rates and miscarriage rates are affected by the presence and the location of uterine fibroids. Analysing the results for the two groups in which a statistically significant difference was found leads to the conclusion that submucosal fibroids have a role in infertility and that removing the submucosal fibroids can improve both the chances of fertilization and pregnancy maintenance [13].

The Cochrane review in its systematic review concluded that a large benefit is potentially seen in hysteroscopically removing submucosal fibroids to improve the chance of clinical pregnancy in women with otherwise unexplained subfertility [6].

8.6 Hysteroscopy in Women with a Uterine Septum

The presence of a malformed uterus can impair normal reproductive performance by increasing the incidence of early and late abortions, preterm deliveries and premature rupture of membranes. However, each type of malformation has a different impact on the pregnancy outcome. Septate uterus is a common congenital uterine malformation. Although clinical studies consistently demonstrate poor obstetric outcomes in patients with a septate uterus, the literature concerning the septate uterus as a fertility factor is controversial. In a review of five studies and nearly 3000 cases, the mean overall incidence of uterine malformation in the general population or the population of fertile women was 4.3 per cent, and out of those, the mean incidence of septate uterus comprised 34.9 per cent

[14]. The mean incidence of Mullerian defects in infertile women was 3.4 per cent, similar to the 4.3 per cent found in the general population of fertile women. This suggests that Mullerian defects have no impact on a woman's fertility. This retrospective review found that a malformed uterus, especially septate uterus, is not a fertility factor, although it may contribute to delayed natural conception in patients with secondary infertility [14].

Mollo and colleagues performed the only prospective controlled trial on patients with a uterine septum and compared the reproductive outcome in 44 patients with unexplained infertility and uterine septum who underwent metroplasty with 134 patients with unexplained infertility and a normal uterine cavity. After one year of follow-up, the pregnancy and live birth rates were significantly higher in patients who underwent removal of a uterine septum than in the group with unexplained infertility and no uterine septum (38.6 per cent vs. 20.4 per cent and 34.1 per cent vs. 18.9 per cent, respectively) [15].

Hysteroscopic septoplasty is the preferred and most common surgical procedure performed for resection of the uterine septum. It is considered a common practice to perform hysteroscopic septoplasty as a therapeutic procedure in patients with recurrent pregnancy loss or a bad obstetric history. Hysteroscopic septoplasty can be performed by using a resectoscope, scissors or laser energy. It is unclear whether the use of a specific instrument improves the outcome. Operative hysteroscopy can be performed by either bipolar or monopolar electrosurgery. When performing hysteroscopic septoplasty by bipolar electrosurgery, a distention medium must be used [16]. The incidence of complications in hysteroscopic septoplasty widely varies depending on the operative procedure and the operator's skills. Sui and colleagues performed 447 hysteroscopic septoplasties and had one case of uterine perforation, six cases of blood loss less than 100 ml and two cases of blood loss >100 ml, three cases of postoperative pelvic infection and five cases of urethral infection, and two cases of bradyardia [17]. In Nouri's pooled analysis of 18 trials, reoperation was required in 6 per cent of the patients [16] These findings suggest that major complications that result from operative hysteroscopic metroplasty are very rare.

Grimbizis and colleagues showed that an untreated septate uterus is associated with increased abortion and preterm delivery rates and reduced term delivery and live birth rates [14]. Mollo and colleagues suggested that in patients with both unexplained infertility and uterine septum, metroplasty might improve pregnancy and term delivery rates [15]. We believe that hysteroscopic metroplasty is mandatory in patients with septate uterus and a bad obstetrical history of spontaneous abortions or preterm delivery. In patients who were diagnosed with unexplained infertility, delayed natural conception and an impaired pregnancy outcome, hysteroscopic metroplasty is justified. Until prospective studies are performed and presented, a more active approach of prophylactic septoplasty rather than a conservative approach should be considered [18].

8.7 The Role of Endometrial Scratch in Improving Endometrial Receptivity

Endometrial scratching (also known as endometrial injury, biopsy or sampling) is currently suggested as a potential treatment to improve endometrial receptivity and thereby pregnancy rates in women undergoing assisted reproductive technology (ART). The most common procedure of endometrial scratching is to perform an endometrial biopsy, with a soft plastic endometrial biopsy catheter such as a Pipelle de Cornier® (Laboratoires C.C.D., France).

In 2000, our group investigated the pattern of endometrial expression of the gap junction protein, Cx43, as a possible parameter for successful implantation. For this purpose, repetitive endometrial samplings were performed during the preceding spontaneous menstrual cycles before IVF treatment in 12 mechanical infertility patients who failed to conceive during several cycles of treatment. Surprisingly, 11 of these patients conceived during the following IVF cycle. After this observation, we conducted a randomized controlled prospective study. We recruited a group of 134 good responder patients who failed to conceive during one or more IVF cycles. Forty-five patients underwent an endometrial biopsy using a Pipelle catheter on days 8, 12, 21 and 26 of the spontaneous menstrual cycle before the IVF-embryo transfer (ET) treatment, and 89 patients underwent IVF treatment without endometrial scratching. Our results showed that transfer of a similar number of embryos resulted in a twofold higher implantation rate (27.7 per cent vs. 14.2 per cent, $p<0.00011$), clinical pregnancy rate (66.7 per cent vs. 30.3 per cent, $p<0.00009$), and live birth rate (48.9 per cent vs. 22.5 per cent, $p<0.016$) in the experimental group as compared to controls [19].

This effect of local endometrial injury was later confirmed by other IVF clinics worldwide [19–24]. Since then, a number of trials in women undergoing ART have investigated the potential fertility enhancing effect of endometrial injury. Several trials have shown a beneficial effect of endometrial injury performed between day 7 of the cycle before stimulation and day 7 of the stimulation cycle [21,23–27], while a few studies could not detect significant improvements [28–30] or even find a negative effect [31]. The Cochrane database systematic reviews conducted a survey to assess the effectiveness and safety of endometrial injury performed before ET in women undergoing ART. They included 14 trials with 1,063 women in the intervention groups and 1,065 women in the control groups. Thirteen studies compared endometrial injury performed between day 7 of the previous cycle and day 7 of the ET cycle versus no injury, and one study compared endometrial injury on the day of oocyte retrieval versus no injury. The results of this survey showed that endometrial injury was associated with an increase in live birth or ongoing pregnancy rates: (RR 1.42, 95 per cent (CI) 1.08 to 1.85; $p= 0.01$). There was no evidence of an effect on miscarriage (RR 0.99, 95 per cent CI 0.63 to 1.53; $p=0.06$) and no effect when comparing endometrial injury on the day of oocyte retrieval versus no injury (RR 0.36, 95 per cent CI 0.18 to 0.71; $p+0.003$). They concluded that endometrial injury performed between day 7 of the previous cycle and day 7 of the ET cycle is associated with an improvement in live birth and clinical pregnancy rates in women with more than two previous ETs [32].

In 2012, Granot and colleagues reviewed the molecular and biochemical evidence that confirms the mechanism by which the injury-induced inflammation improves uterine receptivity and subsequent pregnancy outcomes. They concluded that the local injury generated by an endometrial biopsy increases uterine receptivity by provoking inflammation. Specifically, the findings suggested that an endometrial biopsy provokes an inflammatory response that is probably mediated by tumour necrosis factor-alpha (TNF-α). The pro-inflammatory TNF-α enhances the expression of other cytokines/chemokines that recruit in turn macrophages and dendritic cells (DC) to the site of injury. The injury-induced inflammation also stimulates stem cell-dependent endometrial regeneration [33]. In 2015, the same group performed an in vitro experiment using primary human endometrial cells isolated from the biopsies taken from IVF patients as well as an endometrial cell line. They demonstrated that the injury-induced improved endometrial receptivity in IVF patients with repeated implantation failure is mediated by an inflammatory response that comprises the cooperation between the two endometrial compartments, stromal and epithelial cells. This response is orchestrated by the recruited immune cells, macrophages and DCs. Endometrial biopsies upregulate the expression of pro-inflammatory cytokines that recruit monocytes/macrophages to the site of injury, further inducing their differentiation. This in turn triggers the stromal and epithelial cells to express specific implantation-associated genes, which are involved in the apposition and adhesion of the blastocyst. These events probably do not take place in patients with repeated implantation failures in the absence of the endometrial biopsy treatment [34].

8.8 Summary

Human embryo implantation is a three-stage process that includes apposition, adhesion and invasion. Despite improvements in ovarian stimulation protocols and fertilization procedures, implantation remains the rate-limiting step for successful IVF treatments.

Implantation failure is generally related to inadequate endometrial receptivity in two-thirds of the cases and abnormalities of the embryo in one-third. Many factors can affect the endometrial receptivity and influence the ability of the embryo to implant, such as inappropriate hormonal stimulation, congenital uterine septum, submucosal fibroids, intrauterine adhesions and endometrial polyps.

A routine hysteroscopy does not improve live birth rates in infertile women with a normal transvaginal ultrasound of the uterine cavity scheduled for a first IVF treatment and therefore should not be offered.

Hysteroscopic polypectomy can improve the chance of conceiving in subfertile women with a sonographic diagnosis of endometrial polyps, prior to fertility treatments.

There is a large benefit to hysteroscopically removing submucosal fibroids for improving the chances of a clinical pregnancy in women with otherwise unexplained subfertility.

Hysteroscopic metroplasty is mandatory in patients with septate uterus and a bad obstetrical history of spontaneous abortion or preterm delivery. In patients with incidental finding of a septate uterus and those diagnosed with unexplained infertility, delayed natural conception and impaired pregnancy outcome, hysteroscopic metroplasty is justified.

Endometrial injury performed between day 7 of the previous cycle and day 7 of the ET cycle is associated with improved clinical pregnancy rates and live birth rates in women with more than two previous ETs.

References

1. Taylor E, Gomel V. The uterus and fertility. *Fertility and Sterility* 2008;89: 1–15.

2. Clark TJ, Gupta JK. *Handbook of Outpatient Hysteroscopy. A Complete Guide to Diagnosis and Therapy.* Hodder Education 2005.

3. Campo R, Van Belle Y, Rombauts L, Brosens I, Gordts S. Office mini-hysteroscopy. *Human Reproduction Update* 1999;5: 73–81.

4. Fritz Marc A, Speroff Leon. Clinical Gynecologic Endocrinology and Infertility, 8th Edition. *Lippincott Williams & Wilkins* 2011:1172.

5. Jansen FW, Vredevoogd CB, van Ulzen K et al. Complications of hysteroscopy: a prospective, multicenter study. *Obstetrics and Gynecology* 2000;96: 266–70.

6. Bosteels Jan, Kasius Jenneke, Weyers Steven et al. Hysteroscopy for treating subfertility associated with suspected major uterine cavity abnormalities. *Cochrane Database Systematic Reviews* 2015.

7. National Collaborating Centre for Women's and Children's Health. *Fertility:*

assessment and treatment for people with fertility problems. RCOG Press 2004.

8. Smit JG, Kasius JC, Eijkemans MJC et al. Hysteroscopy before in-vitro fertilisation (inSIGHT): a multicentre, randomised controlled trial. The Lancet, 2016;387, Issue 10038: 2622–9.

9. El-Toukhy T, Campo R, Khalaf Y et al. Hysteroscopy in recurrent in-vitro fertilisation failure (TROPHY): a multicentre, randomised controlled trial. The Lancet, 2016;387, Issue 10038: 2614–1.

10. Silberstein T, Saphier O, van Voorhis BJ, Plosker SM. Endometrial polyps in reproductive-age fertile and infertile women. The Israel Medical Association Journal 2006;8: 192–5.

11. Pérez-Medina T, Bajo-Arenas J, Salazar F et al. Endometrial polyps and their implication in the pregnancy rates of patients undergoing intrauterine insemination: a prospective, randomized study. Human Reproduction 2005;20: 1632–5.

12. Fritz Marc A, Speroff Leon. Clinical Gynecologic Endocrinology and Infertility, 8th Edition. Lippincott Williams & Wilkins 2011: 148–51.

13. Casini ML, Rossi F, Agostini R, Unfer V. Effects of the position of fibroids on fertility. Gynecological Endocrinology 2006;22: 106–9.

14. Grimbizis GF. Camus M, Tarlatzis BC, Bontis JN, Devroey P, Clinical implications of uterine malformations and hysteroscopic treatment results. Human Reproduction Update 2001;7: 161–74.

15. Mollo A, De Franciscis P, Colacurci N et al. Hysteroscopic resection of the septum improves the pregnancy rate of women with unexplained infertility: a prospective controlled trial. Fertility and Sterility 2009;91: 2628–31.

16. Nouri K, Ott J, Huber JC et al. Reproductive outcome after hysteroscopic septoplasty in patients with septate uterus – a retrospective cohort study and systematic review of the literature. Reproductive Biology and Endocrinology 2010;8: 52.

17. Sui L, Wan Q, Zheng RL et al. Transcervical incision of septa: 447 cases. Surg Endosc 2009;23: 2078–84.

18. Or Y, Appelman Z. Is Prophylactic hysteroscopic metroplasty for the septate uterus justified? J Gynecol Surg. 2014;30: 325–8.

19. Raziel A, Schachter M, Strassburger D et al. Favorable influence of local injury to the endometrium in intracytoplasmic sperm injection patients with high-order implantation failure. Fertil Steril. 2007;87: 198–201.

20. Zhou L, Li R, Wang R, Huang HX, Zhong K. Local injury to the endometrium in controlled ovarian hyperstimulation cycles improves implantation rates. Fertil Steril. 2008;89: 1166–76.

21. Karimzadeh MA, Ayazi Rozbahani M, Tabibnejad N. Endometrial local injury improves the pregnancy rate among recurrent implantation failure patients undergoing in vitro fertilisation/intra cytoplasmic sperm injection: A randomised clinical trial. Aust N Z J Obstet Gynaecol. 2009;49: 677–80.

22. Almog B, Shalom-Paz E, Dufort D, Tulandi T. Promoting implantation by local injury to the endometrium. Fertility and Sterility 2010;94: 2026–9.

23. Narvekar SA, Gupta N, Shetty N et al. Does local endometrial injury in the nontransfer cycle improve the IVF-ET outcome in the subsequent cycle in patients with previous unsuccessful IVF?. A randomized controlled pilot study. J Hum Reprod Sci. 2010;3: 15–9.

24. Nastri CO, Teixeira DM, Martins WP. Endometrial injury in the menstrual cycle prior to assisted reproduction techniques to improve reproductive outcomes. Gynecological Endocrinology 2013;25: 401–2.

25. Guven S, Kart C, Unsal M et al. Endometrial injury may increase the clinical pregnancy rate in normoresponders underwent long agonist protocol intracytoplasmic sperm injection cycles with single embryo transfer. Fertil Steril. 2011;96: 277–574.

26. Inal ZHO, Görkemli H, Inal HA. The effect of local injury to the endometrium for implantation and pregnancy rates in ICSI-ET cycles with implantation failure: a randomized controlled study. *European Journal of General Medicine* 2012;9: 223–9.

27. Shohayeb A, El-Khayat W. Does a single endometrial biopsy regimen (S-EBR) improve ICSI outcome in patients with repeated implantation failure? A randomised controlled trial. *European Journal of Obstetrics & Gynecology and Reproductive Biology* 2012;164: 176–9.

28. Karim Zadeh Meybodi M, Ayazi M, Tabibnejad N. Effect of endometrium local injury on pregnancy outcome in patients with IVF/ICSI. *Human Reproduction* 2008;23 (Suppl 1): i126.

29. Safdarian L, Movahedi S, Aleyasine A et al. Local injury to the endometrium does not improve the implantation rate in good responder patients undergoing in-vitro fertilization. *Iranian Journal of Reproductive Medicine* 2011;9: 285–8.

30. Yeung TW, Chai J, Li RH et al. The effect of endometrial injury on ongoing pregnancy rate in unselected subfertile women undergoing in vitro fertilization: a randomized controlled trial. *Human Reproduction* 2014;29: 2474–81.

31. Baum M, Yerushalmi GM, Maman E et al. Does local injury to the endometrium before IVF cycle really affect treatment outcome? Results of a randomized placebo controlled trial. *Gynecological Endocrinology* 2012;28: 933–6.

32. Nastri CO, Lensen SF, Gibreel A et al. Endometrial injury in women undergoing assisted reproductive techniques. *Cochrane Database Syst Rev* 2015;3: CD009517.

33. Granot I, Gnainsky Y, Dekel N. Endometrial inflammation and effect on implantation improvement and pregnancy outcome. *Reproduction*. 2012 December;144: 661–8.

34. Gnainsky Y, Granot I, Aldo P et al. Biopsy-induced inflammatory conditions improve endometrial receptivity: the mechanism of action. *Reproduction* 2015;149: 75–85.

Fibroids and Polyps
Their Effect on Implantation

Beverley Vollenhoven and Sarah Hunt

9.1 Fibroids

Uterine fibroids or leiomyomata are the commonest benign tumours occurring in women of reproductive age. The whirling bundles of smooth muscle cells comprising the myoma are thought to arise from a mutation of a single myometrial cell. Fibroid growth is then mediated by clonal expansion. Approximately 20–50 per cent of women of reproductive age have a symptomatic uterine fibroid [1].

Common presenting symptoms include abnormal uterine bleeding, pain, pressure symptoms and/or subfertility. Symptomatic diagnosis underestimates the true prevalence as some fibroids will be asymptomatic, and symptom onset often precedes reporting and diagnosis by several years. When ultrasound screening studies and pathological data are considered, the incidence of fibroids in premenopausal women is greater than 70 per cent [2, 3]. These estimates include women with increased symptomatology resulting in hysterectomy. Approximately 5–10 per cent of women presenting with infertility will have fibroids; however, it is the likely sole cause of infertility in only 2–3 per cent of women [4].

Fibroids are more common in certain populations. The main risk factors for fibroids are advancing age and race. The incidence rises from puberty to menopause. Hysterectomy specimen data would suggest that the prevalence of fibroids in pre- and postmenopausal women is similar. The incidence of fibroids is two to three times greater in black women as opposed to white women. Women of African ancestry are more likely to develop symptomatic fibroids earlier in reproductive life. They are likely to be larger and result in more symptoms than in women of European descent. Early age of menarche and prenatal diethylstilboestrol (DES) exposure are other hormonal risk factors for fibroid development. Parity and exposure to long-acting progestogens are protective. Lifestyle risk factors include high red meat intake, alcohol consumption and vitamin D deficiency. Diets rich in dairy, fruit and green vegetables reduce the risk of fibroid development [2].

The International Federation of Gynaecology and Obstetrics (FIGO) outlines a numerical classification system for fibroids based on their location within the uterus in proximity to the endometrium (Figure 9.1). It does not reflect the size of fibroids or complexity of disease, but it is hoped that this classification system will result in improved uniformity in the description of fibroids in future clinical trials [5].

The diagnosis of fibroids is reliably made on transvaginal ultrasound. It remains the primary imaging modality in the diagnosis of fibroids due to low cost and patient acceptability (Figure 9.2A). Assessing fibroid location within the uterus is more problematic and inadequate assessment of fibroid location confounds the data in most published fertility studies. Initial studies assessing the sensitivity and specificity of transvaginal ultrasound in

Submucosal	0	Pedunculated intracavity
	1	<50% intramural
	2	≥50% intramural
Other	3	Contacts endometrium, 100% intramural
	4	Intramural
	5	Subserosal, ≥50% intramural
	6	Subserosal, <50% intramural
	7	Subserosal pedunculated
	8	Other (specify e.g. cervical)

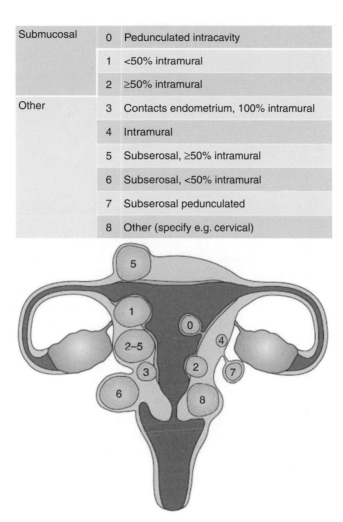

Figure 9.1 Reproduced with permission from REF 2
Source: Adapted from the Korean Medical Association.

the diagnosis of submucosal fibroids showed a high sensitivity and specificity when compared with hysteroscopy. More recent data would suggest lower accuracy, with sensitivity ranges between 69 and 100 per cent and positive predictive value between 47 and 81 per cent [6]. It is also highly operator dependent. Hysterosalpingography is commonly used in infertility evaluation to assess tubal patency and intrauterine contour. It is an inferior examination to transvaginal ultrasound for the diagnosis of fibroids with sensitivity of 50 per cent and specificity 20 per cent [2].

Sonohysterogram, hysteroscopy and magnetic resonance imaging (MRI) are superior modalities for mapping intracavity or submucosal fibroids. Instillation of the cavity with saline (sonohysterography) helps to differentiate small submucous fibroids from the surrounding endometrium and increases the sensitivity and specificity to 89.5 and 100 per cent, respectively (Figure 9.2B) [7]. MRI is significantly more expensive than other imaging

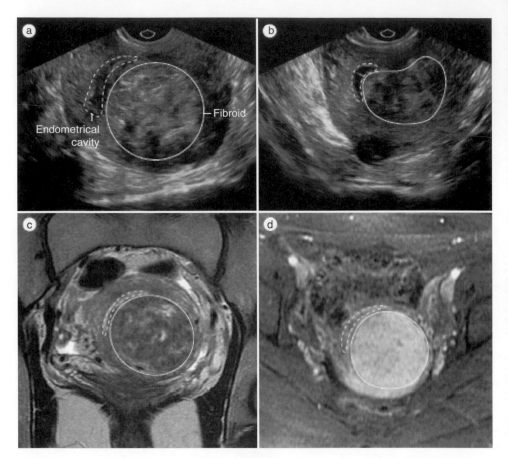

Figure 9.2 **(A)** Transvaginal ultrasonography is the most commonly used imaging modality for the detection of fibroids. A heterogeneous fibroid between 8 and 9 cm in size (solid white border) is seen near the endometrium (dashed white border). **(B)** An intracavitary fibroid (probably FIGO type 2) is seen near the endometrium (dashed white border). **(C)** A T2-weighted MRI scan showing a fibroid (solid white line) on the right and the endometrial cavity (dashed white border) on the left and superior to the fibroids. **(D)** The good blood supply of this fibroid (solid white border) can be visualized in an axial view with intravenous gadolinium-enhanced MRI
Source: Reproduced with permission from REF 2.

modalities but does have a sensitivity and specificity of close to 100 per cent in the diagnosis of fibroids. It is more likely to accurately assess the volume and number of fibroids as compared with ultrasound. It may be of substantial benefit in particular patient groups including those with high body mass index, disease extending beyond the pelvis, those unable to tolerate transvaginal studies or used in preoperative planning (Figure 9.2 C,D) [2].

Hysteroscopy is the gold standard investigation in the diagnosis of submucosal fibroids with sensitivity and specificity of 100 per cent. It carries the risks of an invasive procedure including anaesthetic if required, infection and perforation of the uterus. There is the potential to combine this diagnostic test with a therapeutic procedure if indicated. Hysteroscopy is less accurate in assessing fibroid size and cannot appreciate the myometrial component of L1-2 fibroids [8]. In clinical practice it is rarely performed without pre-operative imaging studies.

The role of fibroids in infertility is controversial. There are several hypotheses to explain the association between fibroids and infertility. These proposed mechanisms include effects on sperm transport, implantation, uterine contractility and endometrial receptivity. [1,4,9,10]

Physical factors relating to the size and location of fibroids may interfere with transport of sperm, oocyte and embryos. Mechanical obstruction of the tubal ostia, oocyte capture, displacement of the cervix and deformity of the uterine cavity may all impact on normal reproductive function [4].

The presence of fibroids also distorts the architecture and normal function of the uterine junctional zone or endomyometrial junction (EMJ). This zone comprises the inner third of the myometrium as it abuts the endometrium. Histologically, there is a reduction in the proportion of endometrial glands overlying leiomyomas. There also appears to be a delay in late secretory endometrial maturation in the presence of fibroids. Uterine peristalsis originates in the EMJ facilitating sperm transport, embryo implantation and menstruation. Directionality of peristalsis changes throughout the menstrual cycle and wave frequency is considerably reduced in the mid-secretory phase, facilitating implantation. Women with fibroids have markedly increased frequency of uterine peristalsis, and this is believed to impair implantation. The EMJ is highly responsive to cyclical changes in oestrogen and progesterone as compared to other myometrial tissue. The presence of fibroids may alter oestrogen and progesterone receptor expression and act to impair decidualization of the endometrium. Decidualization may also be impaired due to reduced EMJ concentrations of macrophages and natural killer (NK) cells in the presence of fibroids [10].

Women with fibroids have dysregulation of a number of factors required for successful implantation. Homeobox gene HOXA10 is responsible for cellular differentiation in the human uterus. Leiomyomas secrete transforming growth factor beta 3 (TGF-β 3), which in turn reduces bone morphogenetic protein 2 (BMP-2) and suppresses HOXA 10. Animal models have demonstrated that reduced or absent HOX10A leads to defective endometrial decidualization and implantation. Women with submucosal fibroids have significantly reduced HOX10A, and women with intramural fibroids have a non-significant trend to reduced HOX10A.

Implantation factor glycodelin promotes angiogenesis and NK cell activity. The level of glycodelin is dynamic through the menstrual cycle with reduced levels seen in the follicular phase and increased levels at the time of implantation. Glycodelin expression appears to be deregulated in women with fibroids. Reduced expression is seen in the secretory phase as compared to non-fibroid controls, likely impairing implantation [1,11].

Blastocyst implantation requires leukaemia inhibitory factor (LIF). Expression of LIF in women with submucous fibroids and endometrial polyps is significantly reduced in the mid-secretory phase as compared to controls [11].

Angiogenesis is vital to successful embryo implantation. Angiogenesis rises rapidly in the early proliferative phase, peaks mid-cycle and then gradually decreases towards the end of the cycle. Adrenomedullin and vascular endothelial growth factor are upregulated in the presence of fibroids and fibroids act as a reservoir for basic fibroblast growth factor (bFGF). It is believed that the presence of increased bFGF concentration in fibroid tissue exerts a paracrine effect impairing implantation in the adjacent myometrium [1,9].

The impact on fibroids and their management in the context of infertility may be considered depending on fibroid location. When fibroids of all locations are considered, women with fibroids have significantly lower implantation, clinical pregnancy and live birth rates and higher rates of spontaneous abortion. Given however that this population is widely heterogeneous, these groups are better considered individually.

9.1.1 Subserosal Fibroids

Systematic review of the available evidence by Pritts et al. demonstrated that there was no evidence that purely subserous fibroid (FIGO L5 to L7) had any detrimental impact on fertility outcomes [6]. Removal of subserosal fibroids is therefore only indicated in symptomatic patients.

9.1.2 Intramural Fibroids

Recent evidence would suggest that fibroids that do not distort the endometrial cavity (L3–L4) still appear to impact on both spontaneous and assisted fertility outcomes. The review by Pritts et al. demonstrated that these women have significantly lower implantation (relative risk (RR) 0.79) and live birth rates (RR 0.78) as well as increased spontaneous miscarriage rates (RR 1.89), compared with non-fibroid controls. There was no significant difference seen in clinical pregnancy rate or preterm delivery [6].

Subsequent meta-analysis by Sunkara et al. showed a 15 per cent reduction in clinical pregnancy rate in women undergoing IVF treatment and a 21 per cent reduction in live birth rate. Pooled analysis of two prospective studies showed a 40 per cent reduction in live birth rate in women with intramural fibroids without cavity distortion [12]. It should be appreciated that significant clinical heterogeneity of the included studies is a weakness of both reviews.

Although there is evidence to suggest that intramural fibroids have a detrimental impact on fertility outcomes, there is no evidence to suggest that myomectomy is of benefit in this population. To date no randomized trial has answered this question; however, observational studies have demonstrated no significant difference in implantation, clinical pregnancy or live birth rate or miscarriage where fibroids do not distort the endometrial cavity [6]. Myomectomy for intramural fibroids cannot therefore be recommended for the management of infertility in an otherwise-asymptomatic patient.

Following comprehensive fertility evaluation, other disorders causing infertility should be treated preferentially to the surgical management of fibroids. In women who are symptomatic of fibroids but desiring future pregnancy, management options are limited. Non-steroidal anti-inflammatory agents (NSAIDs) and tranexamic acid may reduce heavy menstrual bleeding and associated pain [2]. Women with refractory symptoms or symptoms related to fibroid mass may be managed with open or minimally invasive surgery [2].

Abdominal or laparoscopic myomectomy may be associated with significant morbidity including infection, damage to other visceral structures, haemorrhage including blood transfusion and hysterectomy. There is a high rate of postoperative adhesion formation, particularly where a posterior uterine incision is performed. The results of two randomized control trials show that a laparoscopic approach is associated with less post-operative pain, febrile morbidity, smaller mean drop in haemoglobin and shorter length of stay. Cumulative pregnancy rate at 12 months was not significantly different between groups [10]. The rate of uterine rupture in pregnancy or labour following myomectomy is low. Given that it is common clinical practice to recommend caesarean delivery where the uterine cavity has been breached at myomectomy the risk of uterine rupture is likely to be underestimated [13].

Ulipristal acetate, a selective progesterone receptor modulator is now approved for use in the treatment of symptomatic fibroids. Ulipristal treatment is associated with an improvement in menstrual symptoms and regression in fibroid size. The effect on reproductive outcomes of the reduction in fibroid size is at yet unknown. Retrospective analysis of the 21 patients included in the PEARL II and III studies who wished to conceive demonstrated the feasibility of pregnancy following ulipristal therapy. Nineteen patients underwent myomectomy following ulipristal therapy and two patients had near-complete regression of fibroids post treatment. In the group of 21 women, 13 live births were achieved. One live birth resulted from three pregnancies in the two patients who had ulipristal treatment alone. No significant regrowth of fibroids was seen during pregnancy [14]. Ulipristal acetate therapy is not currently recommended for the treatment of women with infertility related to fibroids pending further safety and efficacy data.

Uterine artery embolization is a radiological treatment option for women with large symptomatic fibroids. Embolization of the uterine artery induces temporary ischaemia within the body of the uterus and endometrium, which is intended to be irreversible in the fibroid tissue. The randomized control trial published by Mara and colleagues, evaluated the use of uterine artery embolization or myomectomy for the treatment of intramural fibroids in a population desiring ongoing fertility. Of note, the group randomized to surgical management had significantly higher rates of baseline subfertility than those randomized to embolization. The myomectomy group had significantly greater pregnancy and live birth rates (48 vs. 19 per cent) and lower miscarriage rates. The rate of miscarriage was 64 per cent in the embolization group [15]. It is hypothesized that the transient ischaemia induced in the uterine body may have a detrimental effect on future endometrial function. Furthermore, inadvertent embolization of ovarian tissue may result in premature ovarian insufficiency [16]. Uterine artery embolization should not be recommended over surgical therapy in women desiring future pregnancy and has no current role in the management of infertility associated with fibroids.

Magnetic resonance-guided focused ultrasound surgery (MRgFUS) utilizes MRI to guide ultrasound beams and induce coagulative necrosis in fibroid tissue. Rabinovici and colleagues reported on 54 pregnancies occurring after MRgFUS treatment in 2010, showing 41 per cent live birth rate and 28 per cent miscarriage rate in 51 women [17]. A prospective study examining the role of MrGFUS to improve infertility outcomes has been terminated; the role of this modality remains unclear [18]. The reasons for early termination of this study are unclear; however, past trials of MRgFUS in the United States have encountered issues with low enrolment due to limited insurance coverage.

9.1.3 Submucosal Fibroids

The systematic review conducted by Pritts et al. examined pregnancy outcomes for women with submucous fibroids. This was inclusive of FIGO groups 0–2, patients with any element of cavity distortion. This group demonstrated significantly lower implantation (RR 0.28), clinical pregnancy (RR 0.36) and live birth rates (RR 0.32) as well as significantly higher miscarriage rates (RR 1.68) [6].

Clinical pregnancy rates were significantly higher in women with submucosal fibroids who underwent myomectomy when compared to women where fibroids were untreated. There was no significant difference however in implantation, live birth or miscarriage rates. When compared to infertile women without fibroids, myomectomy resulted in similar implantation, clinical pregnancy, live birth rates and miscarriage rates. This may represent evidence of benefit to treatment given baseline pregnancy outcomes would be expected to be better in this population [6]. A Cochrane review on the role of hysteroscopy in managing subfertility associated with uterine cavity abnormalities assessed the single randomized control trial published by Casini and colleagues. It concluded that there was no evidence of benefit in clinical pregnancy rate for hysteroscopic myomectomy as compared to regular intercourse over a 12-month period (OR2.4, CI 0.97–6.2) [19, 20].

In women with submucous fibroids, a hysteroscopic approach to myomectomy should be performed when indicated. Hysteroscopic myomectomy is associated with a risk of intrauterine adhesion formation of up to 7.5 per cent and a corresponding decrease in reproductive outcomes [10]. This risk must be weighed with the likelihood of improved pregnancy outcome following restoration of the cavity contour.

9.2 Endometrial Polyps

Endometrial polyps are diagnosed in approximately 10–40 per cent of women presenting with abnormal bleeding and 1–12 per cent of women undergoing routine gynaecological examination including transvaginal ultrasound. Women presenting for in vitro fertilization treatment have a relatively high prevalence of endometrial polyps, 32 per cent have such a lesion detected during infertility investigation and treatment [21].

Endometrial polyps consist of benign glands and stroma. They are formed due to proliferation and hypertrophy of the basal layer of the endometrium and their effect on fertility is unclear. Several studies have suggested a deleterious role in implantation; however, the mechanism of this effect is unclear. Hypothesized mechanisms include an associated increase in plasma glycodelin concentrations, gland or stromal resistance to progestogenic stimulation, local inflammatory changes and/or cavity distortion [22].

The diagnosis of endometrial polyp may be suspected on transvaginal ultrasound, hysterosalpingogram or saline infusion sonohysteroscopy. Typical sonographic appearances are of an endogenic mass occupying the uterine lumen surrounded by an echogenic halo. Hysteroscopy remains the gold standard for diagnosis [23]. Polypectomy may be performed by blind polyp avulsion or by resection under vision.

Most studies assessing the effect of endometrial polyps on infertility are observational and results are conflicting. There is only one randomized study assessing the implication of endometrial polyp in infertility. The study by Perez-Medina and colleagues assessed the effect of hysteroscopic polypectomy on pregnancy rates in women undergoing intrauterine insemination. Women who underwent polypectomy were 2.1 times more likely (54 vs. 25.4 per cent) to become pregnant than those who had hysteroscopy and polyp biopsy alone. Of the women who underwent polypectomy, 65 per cent of pregnancies occurred prior to the first IUI cycle suggesting a relationship between the presence of endometrial polyps and infertility [23].

9.3 Summary

The role of fibroids and endometrial polyps in infertility is incompletely understood. Furthermore, the evidence to guide management of infertility patients with fibroids or polyps is poor. The published data consists primarily of observational and largely

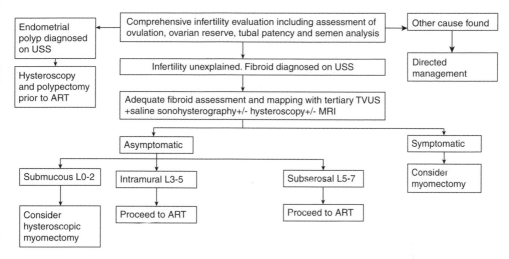

Figure 9.3 Suggested algorithm for the management of fibroids and endometrial polyps in an infertility setting

retrospective studies with conflicting results. A proposed management algorithm is outlined in Figure 9.3.

Subserosal fibroids do not appear to have a detrimental impact on fertility outcomes. In the absence of symptoms, myomectomy in these cases cannot be advocated. Intramural fibroids appear to negatively impact on implantation, live birth and miscarriage rates. Nevertheless, there is insufficient evidence that abdominal or laparoscopic myomectomy improves reproductive outcomes in this population. There is insufficient evidence of safety and benefit to recommend medical or alternative therapies including UAE, MrGFUS and ulipristal at present. Hysteroscopic resection of submucous fibroids and polyps do appear to be of benefit in improving pregnancy outcomes. Further randomized trials in in infertility setting are required to inform management [24].

References

1. Horne AW, Critchley HO. The effect of uterine fibroids on embryo implantation. *Seminars in Reproductive Medicine.* 2007;25(6):483–9.

2. Stewart EA, Laughlin-Tommaso SK, Catherino WH et al. Uterine fibroids. *Nature Reviews Disease Primers.* 2016;2:16043.

3. Cramer SF, Patel A. The frequency of uterine leiomyomas. *American Journal of Clinical Pathology.* 1990;94(4):435–8.

4. Practice Committee of American Society for Reproductive Medicine in collaboration with Society of Reproductive S. Myomas and reproductive function. *Fertility and Sterility.* 2008;90(5 Suppl):S125–30.

5. Munro MG, Critchley HO, Broder MS, Fraser IS, Disorders FWGoM. FIGO classification system (PALM-COEIN) for causes of abnormal uterine bleeding in nongravid women of reproductive age. *International Journal of Gynaecology and Obstetrics: the Official Organ of the International Federation of Gynaecology and Obstetrics.* 2011;113(1):3–13.

6. Pritts EA, Parker WH, Olive DL. Fibroids and infertility: an updated systematic review of the evidence. *Fertility and Sterility.* 2009;91(4):1215–23.

7. Nanda S, Chadha N, Sen J, Sangwan K. Transvaginal sonography and saline infusion sonohysterography in the evaluation of abnormal uterine bleeding. *The Australian & New Zealand Journal*

of Obstetrics & Gynaecology. 2002;42(5): 530–4.

8. Cicinelli E, Romano F, Anastasio PS et al. Transabdominal sonohysterography, transvaginal sonography, and hysteroscopy in the evaluation of submucous myomas. Obstetrics and Gynecology. 1995;85(1):42–7.

9. Makker A, Goel MM. Uterine leiomyomas: effects on architectural, cellular, and molecular determinants of endometrial receptivity. Reproductive Sciences. 2013;20 (6):631–8.

10. Purohit P, Vigneswaran K. Fibroids and infertility. Current Obstetrics and Gynecology Reports. 2016;5:81–8.

11. Pier BD, Bates GW. Potential causes of subfertility in patients with intramural fibroids. Fertility Research and Practice. 2015;1(1):12.

12. Sunkara SK, Khairy M, El-Toukhy T, Khalaf Y, Coomarasamy A. The effect of intramural fibroids without uterine cavity involvement on the outcome of IVF treatment: a systematic review and meta-analysis. Human Reproduction. 2010;25(2):418–29.

13. Guo XC, Segars JH. The impact and management of fibroids for fertility: an evidence-based approach. Obstetrics and Gynecology Clinics of North America. 2012;39(4):521–33.

14. Luyckx M, Squifflet JL, Jadoul P et al. First series of 18 pregnancies after ulipristal acetate treatment for uterine fibroids. Fertility and Sterility. 2014;102(5):1404–9.

15. Mara M, Maskova J, Fucikova Z et al. Midterm clinical and first reproductive results of a randomized controlled trial comparing uterine fibroid embolization and myomectomy. Cardiovascular and Interventional Radiology. 2008;31 (1):73–85.

16. Homer H, Saridogan E. Pregnancy outcomes after uterine artery embolisation for fibroids. The Obstetrician & Gynaecologist. 2009;11(4):265–70.

17. Rabinovici J, David M, Fukunishi H et al. Pregnancy outcome after magnetic resonance-guided focused ultrasound surgery (MRgFUS) for conservative treatment of uterine fibroids. Fertility and Sterility. 2010;93(1):199–209.

18. Health USNIo. ExAblate Treatment of Uterine Fibroids for Fertility Enhancement 2017. Available from: https://clinicaltrials .gov/ct2/show/NCT00730886.

19. Casini ML, Rossi F, Agostini R, Unfer V. Effects of the position of fibroids on fertility. Gynecological Endocrinology: The Official Journal of the International Society of Gynecological Endocrinology. 2006;22(2):106–9.

20. Bosteels J, Kasius J, Weyers S et al. Hysteroscopy for treating subfertility associated with suspected major uterine cavity abnormalities. The Cochrane Database of Systematic Reviews. 2013(1): CD009461.

21. Lieng M, Istre O, Qvigstad E. Treatment of endometrial polyps: a systematic review. Acta obstetricia et gynecologica Scandinavica. 2010;89(8):992–1002.

22. Afifi K, Anand S, Nallapeta S, Gelbaya TA. Management of endometrial polyps in subfertile women: a systematic review. European Journal of Obstetrics, Gynecology, and Reproductive Biology. 2010;151(2): 117–21.

23. Perez-Medina T, Bajo-Arenas J, Salazar F et al. Endometrial polyps and their implication in the pregnancy rates of patients undergoing intrauterine insemination: a prospective, randomized study. Human Reproduction. 2005;20(6): 1632–5.

24. Carranza-Mamane B, Havelock J, Hemmings R et al. The management of uterine fibroids in women with otherwise unexplained infertility. Journal of obstetrics and Gynaecology Canada : JOGC = Journal d'obstetrique et gynecologie du Canada : JOGC. 2015;37(3):277–88.

Chapter 10

Cleavage Stage or Blastocyst Transfer

Which Is Better?

Jason Kasraie

10.1 Introduction

The last 20 years have witnessed a growing debate over the relative advantages and disadvantages of blastocyst (five to six days) versus cleavage stage (two to three days) culture of human embryos, with many publications claiming superiority of one versus the other.

Cleavage stage embryo (see Figure 10.1) transfer dominated the first two decades of human in vitro fertilisation (IVF). This practice was imposed upon the field, as prior to the mid-1990s attempts to culture human embryos to the blastocyst stage met with limited success and tended to be achieved only by co-culture systems. The development of more complex 'sequential' media systems whereby the culture media is changed on day 3 of development to promote blastocyst growth, coupled with a gradual evolution in incubator technology and the growing use of reduced oxygen tension greatly increased blastocyst development and made their transfer in routine IVF viable towards the end of the 1990s [1]. More recently, as our understanding of the needs of the developing embryo has increased, complex single step media has been developed that can also support the routine culture of embryos to the blastocyst stage (see Figure 10.2).

The first two decades of human IVF were characterised by relatively static pregnancy rates. Coupled with this was a belief, probably well founded at the time, that extended

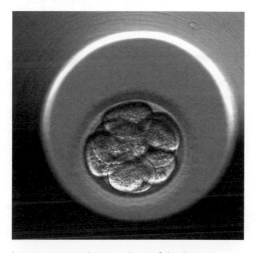

Figure 10.1 A high-quality cleavage stage embryo on day 3 of development

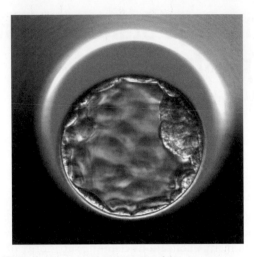

Figure 10.2 A high-quality blastocyst stage embryo on day 5 of development

culture of human embryos in vitro might limit their developmental potential. To put this in context, it is important to understand embryology in the 1980s and 1990s, when understanding and experience was limited. In the last two decades there have been huge advances in ovarian stimulation, cell culture and cryopreservation techniques with concomitant advances in laboratory air quality and environmental control and stabilisation. These advances have led to greater confidence that the environment within laboratories is less likely to be inherently toxic to embryo development. Combined with advances in our understanding of embryo morphokinetic markers, these changes have resulted in huge increases in pregnancy rates per embryo transfer cycle and a decrease in the number of embryos transferred, whilst also making blastocyst culture routine [2]. As the quest to identify the most viable embryo for transfer has continued, blastocyst transfer has increased in popularity as it has been assumed that leaving the embryos to develop in culture for longer will allow more time for selection of the most viable for transfer. Additionally, the international movement to reduce the number of multiple pregnancies through single embryo transfer has been a potent driver for the development of blastocyst culture as the transfer of a single blastocyst has been widely assumed to result in increased implantation and pregnancy rates.

Recently, there has been massive growth in the number of blastocyst transfers worldwide. In the United Kingdom, blastocyst transfers grew from 1 to 47.9 per cent of the total from 2000 to 2014 and the number continues to rise [3].

With the ongoing proliferation of blastocyst transfers, it is important to separate reality from myth and received wisdom or dogma from the reality of the scientific evidence base. This chapter attempts to bring some clarity to the ongoing debate over cleavage stage versus blastocyst transfer.

10.2 What are the Potential Advantages of Blastocyst Transfer?

There are a number of reasons why blastocyst culture might be superior to cleavage stage culture.

10.2.1 Premature Exposure to the Uterine Environment

Having fertilised in the fallopian tube, human embryos do not enter the uterus until the morula stage, on day 4 of development, at the earliest [4]. The fallopian tube and uterus are distinct environments and the constituent components of tubal fluid alter with greater proximity to the uterus. It is hypothesised that the uterus may provide an unnaturally stressful environment for the cleavage stage embryo, thus reducing viability and subsequent pregnancy rates [5].

It has previously been established that humans are rare amongst primate species in the ability of their embryos to survive untimely replacement into the uterus, and without this rare attribute it is likely that human IVF would have taken much longer to develop [6]. It therefore seems rational to argue that blastocysts will gain an advantage simply from being placed into the correct environment at the correct time.

10.2.2 Endometrial Synchronicity

To maximise implantation potential, it is important to synchronise the endometrium to the embryo in order to ensure that the 'window' of endometrial receptivity is open at the time that the blastocyst hatches from the zona pellucida and prepares to implant. It is argued that blastocyst transfer better mimics events in natural conception because the embryo and endometrium are synchronised. It should be noted, however, that super-ovulation in preparation for IVF results in supraphysiological concentrations of oestrogen and progesterone which may alter endometrial development and this in turn may mean that the endometrium is not properly synchronised with the blastocyst in IVF [7]. In short, natural and stimulated cycles likely result in different endometrial hormonal milieu.

10.2.3 Embryo Selection, Increased Implantation and Pregnancy Rates

Cleavage stage embryos are generally assessed using a limited set of morphological and kinetic criteria, which include the number and timing of cell divisions, the evenness of cells and the presence of cellular fragmentation. It is generally accepted that these tools are inadequate at distinguishing euploid embryos with a high implantation potential from aneuploid embryos. A large proportion of morphologically ideal embryos on day 3 are either aneuploid or mosaic, which results in 80–90 per cent implantation failure [8]. Up to day 3 the development of the embryo appears to be controlled primarily by products of maternal DNA. On day 3, compaction occurs and the embryonic genome activates; if this does not occur, the embryo is not viable. Thus, it is argued that extended culture to the blastocyst stage provides an advantage in terms of embryo selection. There is some evidence that blastocyst culture can increase the euploidy rates of transferred embryos; however, aneuploid embryos can reach the blastocyst stage [9]. Critics of blastocyst culture argue that in vitro maturation arrest does not negate in vivo survival and that blastocyst culture risks the loss of some embryos that would have survived to blastocyst in vivo, but do not in vitro because of inadequacies inherent to the in vitro culture environment [7]. Clinical pregnancy rates are higher in fresh blastocyst versus cleavage stage treatments when equal numbers of embryos are transferred [8].

10.2.4 Reduction in Multiple Pregnancy Rates

Multiple pregnancies are associated with significant increases in perinatal mortality and morbidity. There has been an international drive to reduce the number of multiple births from IVF in order to minimise these risks [10]. With higher live birth rates in fresh IVF cycles demonstrated for blastocyst transfer [8], the logical approach has been to encourage blastocyst culture and the transfer of a single blastocyst in high prognosis patients as they are simultaneously more likely to produce blastocysts and are most at risk of multiple pregnancies. This issue is likely to be one of the major drivers for the increase in blastocyst transfer that has been seen in the last decade or so. Whilst the transfer of a single blastocyst will result in a higher pregnancy rate in a fresh embryo transfer, it is not clear whether cumulative pregnancy rates from fresh and frozen embryo transfers are improved. The selection of high prognosis groups might make it less likely that individual patients would not be detrimentally affected by blastocyst culture but there remains the possibility that some embryos might not reach the blastocyst stage in vitro but would have in vivo [7].

10.2.5 Pre-implantation Genetic Diagnosis and Screening

It is now widely accepted that blastocyst trophectoderm biopsy is the most viable technique for obtaining cells for pre-implantation genetic diagnosis (PGD) or pre-implantation genetic screening (PGS) using newly developed technologies such as next-generation sequencing [11]. Thus, blastocyst culture may be the only viable option for patients requiring PGD to reduce transmission of genetically inherited disorders. It should be noted that PGS is still considered to be an unproven and experimental technology by many, and thus culture of embryos to the blastocyst stage for this reason alone is of no proven benefit [12].

10.3 What are the Potential Disadvantages of Blastocyst Transfer?

10.3.1 Cycle Cancellation

Cycle cancellation is significantly higher in blastocyst cycles versus cleavage stage cycles where the patient population is unselected (8.9 vs. 2.8 per cent). This is primarily due to embryo developmental arrest at the cleavage stage. Several studies have demonstrated that women with high yields of oocytes and high-quality eight-cell embryos on day 3 have a greater chance of blastocyst development than those who have no high-quality embryos on day 3 or respond poorly to stimulation [8]. It is strongly advised that patients not classed as 'good prognosis' are counselled regarding these risks [13]. Unfortunately, despite being an area of much research, accurate markers for cleavage stage embryo developmental potential have not been developed, and this makes it extremely difficult to predict which embryos will reach the blastocyst stage in poor prognosis patients. This has led to broad consensus that embryo quality and age should be taken into account when deciding whether to recommend blastocyst transfer to patients [10]. Proponents of blastocyst culture argue that developmentally arrested embryos would probably not have reached the blastocyst stage in any case and it is better not to foster false hope. However, the possibility of a detrimental effect from extended culture cannot be ruled out, [8] and there may be a chance that some embryos would have survived in vivo if transferred to the uterus [7].

10.3.2 Reduced Rates of Embryo Cryopreservation

Patients undergoing blastocyst culture will nearly always have fewer embryos to cryopreserve than they would have had at the cleavage stage, and there is significant evidence to support this. Number of embryos frozen is an important marker of treatment efficacy [8]. Critics of blastocyst transfer highlight that this reduction in overall embryo utilisation has a negative impact on cumulative pregnancy rates and that this would result in further unnecessary oocyte collections, thus increasing risk and cost to the patient [7]. Every embryo frozen represents a future chance of pregnancy. A recent Cochrane systematic review and meta-analysis found no evidence of a difference in cumulative pregnancy rates from cleavage stage versus blastocyst culture, but acknowledged that the quality of the evidence was low and the risk of bias in included studies high, due to the heterogeneity of freezing methods and low number of studies that reported cumulative pregnancy rates from blastocyst cycles [8].

10.3.3 Obstetric and Perinatal Outcomes

Many authors have examined obstetric and perinatal outcomes of pregnancies from blastocyst culture and transfer versus cleavage stage, and this remains a hotly debated topic.

10.3.3.1 Preterm Birth

Early studies suggested an increase in preterm birth rates with blastocyst transfer [14]. More current meta-analyses appear to have confirmed this showing a higher risk of preterm (<37 weeks) and very preterm (<32 weeks) delivery [15]. The authors concede that they were unable to adjust for confounders as the meta-analyses were based on published observational data. A recent commentary has highlighted that several newer studies, not included in the previous meta-analyses, do not agree with their conclusions, arguing that the heterogeneity of culture systems and, pointedly, the lack of consistent practice with regard to low oxygen tension embryo culture is the cause of preterm birth rather than blastocyst culture per se [1].

10.3.3.2 Monozygotic Twinning

There is an increased risk of twinning inherent to the transfer of more than one embryo in IVF procedures. There is also an increase in the risk of monozygotic twinning, which results from the fission of a single early embryo and the formation of two foetuses. The monozygotic twinning rate has been reported as being higher for blastocyst versus cleavage stage embryos. Approximately 1 in 330 spontaneous pregnancies results in the birth of monozygotic twins, rates after cleavage stage transfer in IVF are around 1 per cent [2], whilst the transfer of blastocysts is reported to result in a two- to threefold increase in the rate over this [7]. Monozygotic pregnancies are the highest risk multiple pregnancies and are associated with significant levels of perinatal and obstetric morbidity. Significant fetal complications of monozygotic twinning include intra-uterine growth restriction, preterm delivery, twin-to-twin transfusion syndrome, conjoined twins, microsomia, acardia and congenital talipes equinovarus. Maternal complications include pre-eclampsia, gestational hypertension and gestational diabetes [2, 16]. There are several potential mechanisms for increased monozygotic twinning in blastocyst transfer; these include extended culture per se, zona pellucida tampering leading to herniation of the blastomeres

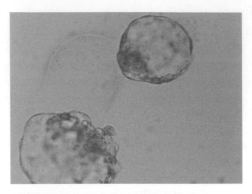

Figure 10.3 Monozygotic twinning caught on camera. Two blastocysts form when hatching from a single zona pellucida on day 6. Note the presence of two distinct inner cell masses which have just split from each other

(e.g. ICSI or assisted hatching) (see Figure 10.3) and ovarian stimulation [16]. Alternatively, developmental dissonance between individual cells might result in early expulsion and fission of the embryo [8].

The link between blastocyst transfer and monozygotic twinning is not certain however, and other studies have noted no increase [13], citing that there is heterogeneity in culture media and systems used or that studies to date have been retrospective, small or poorly designed which makes it difficult to draw a definitive conclusion. When comparing randomised controlled trials in a systematic review and meta-analysis, one group concluded that there was no difference in monozygotic twinning rates between cleavage stage and blastocyst culture. Another study, which controlled for embryo cohort quality also found no difference [17]. It should be noted that there may be detection bias associated with more rigorous assessment of zygosity amongst twins that are conceived through assisted conception, whilst the fact that genetic testing is necessary to detect over 40 per cent of cases may mean that there is significant under-reporting of monozygotic twinning rates [2].

10.3.3.3 Congenital Anomalies

The background risk of congenital anomalies for naturally conceived infants is 3–5 per cent. IVF alone is associated with a 30–40 per cent increased risk of major congenital anomalies when adjusting for confounding factors such as multiple births. This increased risk is thought to be attributable in part to the infertility of those being treated, as couples taking longer than 12 months to conceive and who do not undergo IVF also have an increased risk of congenital anomaly [18]. A recent systematic review and meta-analysis concluded there were significantly higher odds of congenital anomaly with blastocyst stage transfer versus cleavage stage [19]. However, a recent population based registry study from Sweden found no increase in risk of birth defects after blastocyst transfer [20]. Some have argued that under good laboratory conditions, with low oxygen tension culture, there appears to be no detrimental effect on the health of offspring from blastocyst culture [1]. Again this would appear to be a case where confounding factors and the sheer heterogeneity of culture media, systems and practice in IVF means that the truth of the matter is difficult to elucidate (see Figure 10.4).

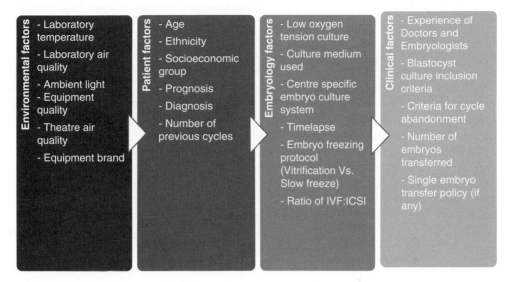

Figure 10.4 Heterogeneity in assisted conception practice – why we are not comparing like with like when we compare blastocyst transfer and cleavage stage transfer results from different centres

10.3.3.4 Genetic Abnormalities (Imprinting)/Large for Gestational Age Babies

There is considerable interest in the long-term consequences of assisted conception on the genome. Epigenetic changes are alterations to the parts of the genome that are not contained in the DNA sequence alone and regulation of these epigenetic aspects of the genome are pivotal to many parts of genome function. These epigenetic changes include nucleosome remodelling, histone modification, higher-order chromatin reorganisation, non-coding RNA regulation and DNA methylation. Several studies have linked IVF to changes in DNA methylation and the frequency of epigenetic alterations to the chromosomes. Imprinting is a key embryo developmental process and describes the method through which genes are epigenetically expressed and regulated [21].

Epigenetic changes related to DNA methylation are the most studied in clinical IVF and include disorders such as Angelman, Beckwith-Wiedemann and Silver-Russell syndromes, all of which seem to appear in increased numbers in IVF children. Normally imprinted genes demonstrate 'parent-of origin' differences in allelic expression, whereby one allele's expression is restricted whilst the other allele is in an inactivated state [22]. Many genes identified thus far as being imprinted regulate growth pre-and/or postnatally. Several mechanisms have been proposed for an increase in epigenetic alteration in IVF including manipulation of sperm, ovarian stimulation, oocyte retrieval and, importantly for blastocyst culture, duration of embryo culture. A recent systematic review and meta-analysis [21] concluded that there is a significant association between ART and imprinting disorders but there is no evidence of generalised changes in the DNA methylation of studied genes. It is important to note that the underlying rate of imprinting disorders remains low, with the overall combined risk of Beckwith-Wiedemann, Angelman and Silver-Russell syndrome in children born from assisted conception being approximately 1 in 5000. Whilst embryo culture per se has been implicated in an increase in imprinting disorders, there is no strong evidence that extended culture increases the underlying risk. One recent study found perturbed imprinted methylation in 76 per cent of cleavage stage embryos and 50 per cent of blastocysts, although the numbers included in the study are too low to conclude that blastocyst culture reduces the risk of imprinting disorders [22]. Finally, it has been suggested that infertile couples have an increased risk of imprinting disorder per se and that this may be a major confounding factor when examining the effect of IVF and embryo culture on their incidence. However, a recent systematic review and meta-analysis [21] was unable to compare DNA methylation levels and the risk of epigenetic and imprinting disorders in children born spontaneously to fertile couples versus infertile couples as no papers were identified that met reasonable inclusion criteria.

Large for gestational age babies have been reported to result from blastocyst culture [7]; however, at this time there are considerable limitations to the studies that have been performed and a consensus view has not emerged. It should be noted that IVF has most often been associated with small for gestational age offspring, and there are reported differences in birth weights of babies born from culture in different media types and brands. As with other claimed disadvantages to blastocyst culture, the sheer heterogeneity of practice in the field makes it extremely difficult to rule out confounders.

10.3.3.5 Miscarriage

Although some authors have claimed an increased (and occasionally a decreased) risk of miscarriage from blastocyst transfer, a systematic review and meta-analysis produced by the Cochrane collaboration did not find any difference in miscarriage rates between cleavage stage embryo transfer and blastocyst transfer [8]. Similar results have been found by systematic reviews and meta-analyses from other groups [2], making it highly likely that there is no increase in miscarriage rates with blastocyst culture and transfer.

10.3.4 Altered Sex Ratio

The reported normal sex ratio at birth of spontaneously conceived offspring is 1.05:1.00 for male and female, respectively. There have been several reports that blastocyst transfer leads to an altered sex ratio in favour of the male [7]. A systematic review and meta-analysis [23] found that 56.8 per cent versus 50.9 per cent of offspring were males for blastocyst and cleavage stage transfer, respectively. Although the exact mechanism for this skewed sex ratio is yet to be elucidated, it is considered most likely to be an artefact of current embryo selection techniques. Male embryos appear to develop faster and thus contain a greater number of cells on average at any given time. Because embryo selection is based on morphokinetic algorithms and blastocysts for transfer are selected on the basis of cell number and expansion status, it thus becomes more likely that male embryos will be selected for transfer, with this trend being exacerbated at later stages of development.

10.4 Discussion

On the surface, blastocyst transfer appears to offer some advantages over traditional cleavage stage transfer (see Figure 10.5). Fresh blastocyst transfer may result in increased live birth rates per couple or woman, and clinical pregnancy rates appear to be higher in fresh blastocyst transfer when equal numbers of embryos are transferred.

Extended culture may offer the opportunity for the transfer of embryos with the greatest implantation potential as they effectively self-select by surviving the rigours of five to six days of in vitro culture. Conversely, extended culture may result in the unnecessary

---

Advantages of blastocyst transfer

- Increased pregnancy rate per fresh embryo transfer when equal numbers of embryos transferred
- Can be used in next-generation PGD
- Assists in the selection of a single embryo for transfer and can be used to reduce the risk of multiple birth

Unclear/not enough evidence available

- More information required on differences with cleavage stage transfer in cumulative pregnancy rates
- Monozygotic twinning rates
- Rates of congenital anomaly
- Imprinting errors/large for gestational age offspring

Disadvantages of blastocyst transfer

- Increased cycle cancellation rate
- Altered sex ratio (favours males)
- Reduction in embryo cryopreservation rates
- Preterm birth rates

Figure 10.5 A synopsis of available evidence for advantages and disadvantages of blastocyst versus cleavage stage transfer

abandonment of treatments and may not give all embryos the opportunity to develop to their full potential in the challenging in vitro culture environment, and we simply do not know if all embryos that fail to reach the blastocyst stage in vitro would do so in vivo.

Transfer of blastocysts may place them into a more welcoming uterus with a synchronised endometrium; however, it may not be necessary for the human embryo to be placed into a synchronised environment and the hormonal milieu, and thus development of the endometrium may be altered by superovulation regimes, so endometrial synchrony as a justification for blastocyst culture may be unfounded.

An argument for increased implantation rates is often used for blastocyst transfer; however, implantation rate may be a poor outcome parameter, and it has been argued that it should be abandoned from infertility research. This is particularly pertinent when comparing outcomes from groups where different numbers of embryos are often transferred as in this case [24]. The largest systematic review and meta-analysis of the subject to date concluded that implantation data would not generate valid estimates due to the unit of analysis used [8].

Increasingly, there is a move to consider cumulative live birth rates from a single oocyte collection as the most useful measure of treatment success. It is difficult to gather true cumulative data (i.e. comparative data from fresh and all frozen embryos from a single oocyte collection) as there are often long delays between embryo cryopreservation and use, and frequently frozen embryos are not used if a pregnancy ensues. Nevertheless, some authors have attempted to compare blastocyst and cleavage stage transfer with this measure. Embryo utilisation rates (the number of embryos that are transferred or frozen and subsequently transferred) are lower in blastocyst culture due to embryo developmental arrest in vitro. The number of treatment cancellations is also significantly higher [8], which can be devastating for patients. Proponents of blastocyst culture argue that if an embryo does not reach the blastocyst stage in vitro, then it would not in vivo; and thus if a cycle is cancelled, we avoid giving patients false hope.

In theory, cumulative pregnancy rates offer a way to test this in vitro survival hypothesis because, if it is true, there should be no difference between blastocyst and cleavage stage cumulative success. Many authors have observed higher cumulative pregnancy rates for cleavage stage transfer overall and others have reported that cumulative pregnancy rates in the cleavage stage group equalled those in the blastocyst group (thus eliminating the advantage from blastocyst transfer in fresh cycles). One group saw an increase in cumulative pregnancy rates for women 35 or older with >4 zygotes collected [25], which may have been due to their use (and success with) vitrification for the cryopreservation of blastocysts. Thus, a clear conclusion on cumulative pregnancy rates remains elusive, and whilst the weight of published evidence appears to support a superior outcome with cleavage stage transfer, difficulties with cryo-survival of blastocysts may be a confounding factor.

With higher pregnancy rates per fresh embryo transfer, blastocysts appear to offer an ideal way to minimise the risk of multiple pregnancy whilst not decreasing the chance of pregnancy in high prognosis patients. This is perhaps the most logical argument for blastocyst culture, as it appears to reduce risk to the patient and offspring without an obvious negative effect. Properly designed algorithms are necessary to ensure low treatment failure rates [10] with the aim that no individual who would have achieved a live birth through double embryo transfer remains childless through single embryo transfer.

It does appear that blastocyst culture is disadvantageous in terms of increased cycle cancellation rates, decreased embryo utilisation rates, alterations in sex ratios and increases in preterm birth.

There may be an increase in congenital anomalies and monozygotic twinning rates but the data on this is sparse or contradictory, and when confounding factors are taken into account, it is difficult to reach a definitive conclusion. There is no clear difference in miscarriage rates or genetic abnormalities (including imprinting errors).

A major problem in investigating the differences between cleavage stage and blastocyst culture is the sheer heterogeneity of the culture media, stimulation regimes, treatment regimes and laboratory culture systems that are used. This makes it extremely difficult for systematic reviews and meta-analyses to draw firm conclusions. It is also important to consider the enormous contrast in reported rates of blastulation in the literature, which can vary from 20 to 60 per cent and serve as a stark illustration of the differences in practice inherent to the field [8]. There are, of course, different ways to approach a problem, and a centre with high blastulation rates may have these purely through patient selection or differences in reporting.

There has been enormous proliferation in the number of blastocyst cycles that are undertaken. The transfer of a single blastocyst can significantly decrease the risk of twins whilst maintaining an acceptable pregnancy rate in fresh cycles. Another driver for blastocyst culture and transfer may be purely commercial; in most countries, assisted conception clinics are judged on their live birth rate per fresh cycle of treatment. Clinics may therefore be perversely incentivised to culture to the blastocyst stage in order to select patients with the highest prognosis. In a system where any cancelled cycles of treatment are not taken into account, a clinic may quite easily appear exceptional in terms of pregnancy rate per cycle simply by always trying to culture to the blastocyst stage and cancelling any cycles where embryos do not reach the blastocyst stage.

10.5 Conclusions

The question of whether blastocyst culture represents a true paradigm shift in the field is yet to be answered, and it is likely that the truth of the matter is nuanced rather than clear-cut, being dependent upon the analysis of multiple factors and upon individual patient characteristics.

If a couple are good prognosis and at high risk of twinning, then it is probably preferable to culture to the blastocyst stage in order to transfer a single blastocyst and minimise the risk of twins. This approach may result in a lower embryo utilisation rate but on balance risk reduction and the maximisation of pregnancy rates in the fresh cycle may make it worthwhile. Likewise, there might be specific situations where a pre-existing medical condition in the female (regardless of age) warrants the transfer of a single blastocyst to minimise the risk of twinning. If PGD is necessary, then blastocyst culture is certainly warranted.

Older couples with a reduced chance of blastocyst formation in vitro might benefit from the transfer of two cleavage stage embryos in a fresh cycle and the cryopreservation of all other viable embryos in order to maximise embryo utilisation and cumulative pregnancy rate. This approach would ensure every embryo has the opportunity to reach the blastocyst stage in the potentially more clement environment of the uterus.

It is important to understand that blastocyst culture, whilst beneficial in some instances, cannot be considered a panacea at this stage. Differences in practice and environment between centres mean that what works for some may not work for others. It is for individual centres to determine treatment algorithms that best benefit their patients, and it is likely at this time that these algorithms should include a mixture of cleavage stage and blastocyst transfer.

So which is better? Couples should be properly counselled over the relative advantages and disadvantages of blastocyst versus cleavage stage transfer. Ultimately, the decision must be based around the balance between the need to achieve a pregnancy *now*, in which case the transfer of a fresh blastocyst is advantageous against the need to maximise cumulative pregnancy rates, and reduce the requirement for further expensive and risky oocyte collections. Blastocyst transfer is better in some circumstances, cleavage stage transfer in others.

It seems sensible to conclude that there remains a pressing need for large high-quality prospective randomised trials with cumulative pregnancy as an endpoint in order to address the question of embryo utilisation and finally determine whether blastocyst culture is disadvantageous to couples in this respect whilst also clarifying whether some embryos are disadvantaged by blastocyst culture.

References

(1) Gardner DK. The impact of physiological oxygen during culture, and vitrification for cryopreservation, on the outcome of extended culture in human IVF. *Reproductive BioMedicine Online*, 2016, Volume 32, Issue 2, 137–141.

(2) Johnson N, Blake D, Farquhar C. Blastocyst or cleavage-stage embryo transfer? *Best Practice & Research Clinical Obstetrics & Gynaecology*, 2007, Volume 21, Issue 1, 21–40.

(3) The Human Fertilisation and Embryology. Fertility Treatment in 2014: Trends and Figures. Authority (www.hfea.gov.uk/10243.html).

(4) Croxatto HB, Fuentealba B, Diaz S, Pastene L, Tatum HJ. A simple nonsurgical technique to obtain unimplanted eggs from human uteri. *American Journal of Obstetrics & Gynecology*, 1972, Volume 112, Issue 5, 662–668.

(5) Munné S, Sandalinas M, Escudero T, Márquez C, Cohen J. Chromosome

mosaicism in cleavage-stage human embryos: evidence of a maternal age effect. *Reproductive BioMedicine Online*, 2002, Volume 4, Issue 3, 223–232.

(6) Marston JH, Penn R, and Sivelle PC. Successful autotransfer of tubal eggs in the rhesus monkey (Macaca mulatta). *J Reprod Fertil*, 1977, Volume 49, Issue 1, 175–176.

(7) Maheshwari A, Hamilton M, Bhattacharya S. Should we be promoting embryo transfer at blastocyst stage? *Reproductive BioMedicine Online*, 2016, Volume 32, Issue 2, 142–146.

(8) Glujovsky D, Farquhar C, Quinteiro Retamar AM, Alvarez Sedo CR, Blake D. Cleavage stage versus blastocyst stage embryo transfer in assisted reproductive technology. *Cochrane Database of Systematic Reviews*, 2016, Issue 6.

(9) Staessen C, Platteau P, Van Assche E et al. Comparison of blastocyst transfer with or without preimplantation genetic diagnosis for aneuploidy screening in couples with advanced maternal age: a prospective randomized controlled trial. *Hum Reprod* 2004, Volume 19, Issue 12, 2849–2858.

(10) Harbottle S, Hughes C, Cutting R, Roberts S, Brison D, and On Behalf Of The Association Of Clinical Embryologists & The (ACE) British Fertility Society (BFS). Elective single embryo transfer: an update to UK best practice guidelines. *Hum Fertil (Camb).* 2015 Sep;18(3):165–83.

(11) Dahdouh EM, Balayla J, García-Velasco JA. Impact of blastocyst biopsy and comprehensive chromosome screening technology on preimplantation genetic screening: a systematic review of randomized controlled trials. *Reproductive BioMedicine Online*, 2015, Volume 30, Issue 3, 281–289.

(12) Gleicher N, Kushnir VA, Barad DH. Preimplantation genetic screening (PGS) still in search of a clinical application: a systematic review. *Reprod Biol Endocrinol.* 2014 Mar 15;12:22.

(13) The Practice Committees of the American Society for Reproductive Medicine and the Society for Assisted Reproductive Technology. Blastocyst culture and transfer in clinical-assisted reproduction: a committee opinion. *Fertility and Sterility*, 2013, Volume 99, Issue 3, 667–672.

(14) Schwärzler P, Zech H, Auer M et al. Pregnancy outcome after blastocyst transfer as compared to early cleavage stage embryo transfer. *Hum Reprod* 2004, Volume 19, Issue 9, 2097–2102.

(15) Maheshwari A, Kalampokas T, Davidson J, Bhattacharya S. Obstetric and perinatal outcomes in singleton pregnancies resulting from the transfer of blastocyst-stage versus cleavage-stage embryos generated through in vitro fertilization treatment: a systematic review and meta-analysis. *Fertility and Sterility*, 2013, Volume 100, Issue 6, 1615–1621.e10.

(16) Sharara FI, Abdo G. Incidence of monozygotic twins in blastocyst and cleavage stage assisted reproductive technology cycles. *Fertility and Sterility*, 2010, Volume 93, Issue 2, 642–645.

(17) Franasiak JM, Dondik Y, Molinaro TA et al. Blastocyst transfer is not associated with increased rates of monozygotic twins when controlling for embryo cohort quality. *Fertility and Sterility*, 2015, Volume 103, Issue 1, 95–100.

(18) The British Fertility Society and the Royal College of Obstetricians & Gynaecologists. Scientific Impact Paper No. 8. In Vitro Fertilisation: Perinatal Risks and Early Childhood Outcomes. May 2012. www.rcog.org.uk/globalassets/documents/guidelines/scientific-impact-papers/sip_8.pdf

(19) Dar S, Lazer T, Shah PS, Librach CL. Neonatal outcomes among singleton births after blastocyst versus cleavage stage embryo transfer: a systematic review and meta-analysis. *Hum Reprod Update* 2014, Volume 20, Issue 3, 439–448.

(20) Ginstrom-Ernstad E, Bergh C, Khatibi A et al. Neonatal and maternal outcome after blastocyst transfer: a

population-based registry study. *American Journal of Obstetrics & Gynecology*, 2016, Volume 214, Issue 3, 378.e1–378.e10.

(21) Lazaraviciute G, Kauser M, Bhattacharya S, Haggarty P, Bhattacharya S. A systematic review and meta-analysis of DNA methylation levels and imprinting disorders in children conceived by IVF/ICSI compared with children conceived spontaneously. *Hum Reprod Update* 2014, Volume 20, Issue 6, 840–852.

(22) White CR, Denomme MM, Tekpetey FR et al. High Frequency of Imprinted Methylation Errors in Human Preimplantation Embryos. Scientific Reports 5, Article number: 17311 (2015).

(23) Chang HJ, Lee JR, Jee BC, Suh CS, Kim SH. Impact of blastocyst transfer on offspring sex ratio and the monozygotic twinning rate: a systematic review and meta-analysis. *Fertility and Sterility*, 2009, Volume 91, Issue 6, 2381–2390.

(24) Griesinger G. Beware of the 'implantation rate'! Why the outcome parameter 'implantation rate' should be abandoned from infertility research. *Hum Reprod* 2016, Volume 31, Issue 2, 249–251.

(25) Fernández-Shaw S, Cercas R, Braña C, Villas C, Pons I. Ongoing and cumulative pregnancy rate after cleavage-stage versus blastocyst-stage embryo transfer using vitrification for cryopreservation: Impact of age on the results. *J Assist Reprod Genet* (2015), Volume 32, 177.

Dummy Embryo Transfer

Khaldoun Sharif and Gamal I. Serour

11.1 Introduction

Embryo transfer (ET) is the final hurdle in the in vitro fertilisation (IVF) treatment process. Up to that step, most patients starting IVF achieve successful pituitary desensitisation, ovarian stimulation, egg collection, fertilisation and embryo cleavage, with about 80 per cent reaching the stage of ET. However, the chance of an embryo implanting after transfer is no more than 10–20 per cent on average. This relative inefficiency has been apparent since the early days of IVF, when Steptoe and Edwards described ET as 'the weakest part of our technique' [1]. Those pioneers have also recognised the fact that when there was a technical difficulty in passing the transfer catheter through the cervix, it resulted in a reduction in the pregnancy rate [1]. A recent meta-analysis of controlled studies has shown this reduction to be highly significant (OR=0.64 (95% CI 0.52–0.77)) [2]. A study of more than 7,000 ETs demonstrated that a technically difficult ET is associated with a reduced pregnancy rate [3].

The incidence of difficult ET is generally about 10 per cent of all transfers, ranging from the slightly difficult to the impossible. In a report by Wood and colleagues in 1985 [4] of 867 ETs, 5.6 per cent were reported as difficult (requiring manipulation in and out to introduce the catheter), 3.2 per cent were reported as very difficult (requiring manipulation for over five minutes or cervical dilatation) and 1.3 per cent were impossible to perform [4]. Additionally, it has been demonstrated that each additional manoeuvre needed to transfer the embryos leads to a progressive reduction in the pregnancy rate [3]. Research into improving the results of the ET procedure addressed several techniques on how best to perform ET. The use of dummy embryo transfer (Dummy ET) had been proposed as a possible pre-transfer procedure to improve the outcome of ET.

11.2 Dummy Embryo Transfer

Dummy (or 'mock' or 'trial', as called by some groups) ET is a transfer procedure performed with an empty catheter, as a form of 'rehearsing' the real procedure [5–7]. It allows the practitioner to assess the anticipated ease or difficulty with which the real transfer will be met and plan any necessary steps needed to make it easier. When Dummy ET is performed, the operator can get information on the length and direction of the uterine cavity, the utero-cervical angle and the most suitable transfer catheter to be used for ET. The malleable transfer catheter at the time of ET can be shaped accordingly in order to minimise the risk of a difficult transfer. Dummy ET has been shown to be a useful tool in clinical practice, in researching the ET process and in training healthcare providers on the technique of ET.

11.3 Dummy Embryo Transfer in Clinical Practice

A randomised controlled trial (involving 335 patients) of Dummy ET performed by Mansour and colleagues during the month before the start of the IVF cycle has shown that Dummy ET assisted in the choice of the most suitable catheter to use in the real transfer, reduced the incidence of difficult transfers and significantly improved implantation and pregnancy rates [5].

In that trial, Dummy ET was performed as an 'interval' procedure (i.e. during a non-treatment cycle) [5]. However, as the uterus is a mobile organ, its position can be different between the time of the interval mock transfer and the real transfer, particularly if it was retroverted. Furthermore, the Dummy ET is performed during a non-stimulated cycle when the uterus and the cervix are not exposed to the same hormonal milieu as at the time of the true ET. In a study involving 996 ET procedures, the position of the retroverted uterus at the time of the interval dummy transfer changed to anteverted in 55 per cent of cases at the time of the real transfer [8]. Therefore, other groups have performed the dummy transfer at different times, such as day 6 of ovarian stimulation [9], at oocyte retrieval [10] and immediately before the real transfer [11]. Some have voiced concern about immediate pre-real transfer Dummy ET on the basis that it may be detrimental to the outcome, perhaps because of possible initiation of uterine contractions or injury to the endometrium with no time for healing. Torre and colleagues found that Dummy ET did not affect uterine contractility [12]. Allahbadia GN and colleagues in a comparative study found that the pregnancy outcome, in IVF cycles with trial Dummy ET done one month prior to cycle versus those done on the day of ET, was the same [13]. One may conclude that the timing of the dummy transfer is an individual operational decision for each IVF programme to make.

11.4 Dummy Embryo Transfer as a Research Tool

The performance of Dummy ET helps in better understating and refining of the ET procedure. It allows researchers to safely investigate the potential effects of different conditions and interventions on ET, without jeopardising real embryos. A radiopaque dye was used with Dummy ET to study the rate of uterine expulsion of the injected dye. The rate of expulsion of the dye in the Fallopian tubes, the cervix and the vagina was 38.2 per cent, 8.8 per cent and 11.8 per cent, respectively, suggesting the mechanism for the occurrence of ectopic pregnancy or the loss of embryos in IVF [14]. Dummy ET using echo dense solution was used to investigate the effect of a difficult transfer (mimicked by touching the uterine fundus) on the uterine activity and relocation of the transferred solution. It was found that easy Dummy ET did not change myometrial contractile activity, and the transferred solution remained in the upper part of the uterine cavity. On the other hand, a difficult procedure generated strong random waves in the fundal area and waves from fundus to cervix, which relocated the solution in six out of seven cases. In four cases the transferred bolus moved from the upper part of the uterus towards the cervix and in two cases into Fallopian tubes, suggesting a mechanism by which a difficult transfer can lead to a lower pregnancy rate [15]. The potential for uterine contraction relocating the transferred fluid was also confirmed by other investigators using Dummy ET [16].

Other factors that were investigated by the use of Dummy ET and found to affect the chances of uterine retention of the transferred solution are viscosity of the fluid and the volume of air it contained. The more similar the viscosity was to the uterine fluid and the less air it contained, the higher the chances of retention [17].

Dummy ET was used to investigate the effect of applying a tenaculum to the cervix. It was found that applying a tenaculum to the cervix increased uterine junctional zone contractions and is thus best avoided at the time of ET [18]. Dummy ET was also used to assess the influence of the position and length of the uterus on implantation and clinical pregnancy rates in IVF cycles [19].

11.5 Dummy ET as a Training Tool

The pregnancy rate after ET has been shown to be different between members of the same practice using similar techniques, and this may be related to the experience and dexterity of each individual practitioner [20]. This is also highly suggested by the finding that trainees in reproductive medicine usually need to perform about 50 ETs to achieve a similar pregnancy rate to those more experienced members of the same IVF programme [21]. Therefore, the question for training programmes is: How to reach this adequate proficiency level for trainees without adversely affecting the pregnancy rate in each individual patient, who rightly deserves and demands an optimal ET outcome [22]?

Programmes usually use training in intra-uterine insemination (IUI) as a 'stepping-stone' towards ET, but this has been found to be inadequate. A study comparing trainees for ET who have had training in IUI with their colleagues who have not had such training found no difference in the pregnancy rate during the learning period [23].

An appropriate method for training in ET is the use of Dummy ET by the trainee in the presence of the experienced practitioner [22]. Not only can this provide experience for the trainee without affecting the pregnancy rate, but the stress of the real patient scenario may provide a more realistic experience for the trainee, as opposed to training on a simulator [22]. This method has been used to train physicians and nurses in ET, with both groups achieving proficiency without affecting the pregnancy rate [24].

Another training strategy that utilises Dummy ET is the use of the 'afterloading' method [25]. In this technique, the trainee performs an immediate Dummy ET at the time of ET. If the catheter passes easily into the uterus, the trainee simply leaves the outer sheath of the catheter in place and loads the embryos into a second inner catheter to be loaded in the already-inserted outer sheath of the dummy catheter. This differs from a simple dummy transfer, because once access to the endometrial cavity is achieved, there is no additional step of catheter removal and replacement [22,25].

11.6 Conclusion

ET, although technically easy in most cases, may be difficult, which can result in a lower pregnancy rate. The use of Dummy ET, when the procedure is rehearsed with no embryos, has been shown to minimise the risk of a difficult transfer and increases implantation and pregnancy rates. It is also a useful tool in training for ET and in increasing our understanding of the procedure.

References

1. Steptoe PC, Edwards RG, Purdy JM. Clinical aspects of pregnancies established with cleaving embryos grown in vitro. *J Obstet Gynaecol* 1980; 87:757–68.

2. Agameya A-F, Sallam HN. Does a difficult embryo transfer affect the results of IVF and ICSI? A meta-analysis of controlled studies. *Fertil Steril* 2014; 101:e8.

3. Kava-Braverman A, Martínez F, Rodríguez I et al.. What is a difficult transfer? Analysis of 7,714 embryo transfers: the impact of maneuvers during embryo transfers on pregnancy rate and a proposal of objective assessment. *Fertil Steril* 2017; 3:657–63.

4. Wood C, McMaster R, Rennie G, Trounson A, Leeton J. Factors influencing pregnancy rates following in vitro fertilization and embryo transfer. *Fertil Steril* 1985; 43:245–50.

5. Mansour R, Aboulghar M, Serour G. Dummy embryo transfer: a technique that minimizes the problems of embryo transfer and improves pregnancy rate in human in vitro fertilization. *Fertil Steril* 1990; 54: 678–81.

6. Sharif K, Afnan M, Lenton W. Mock embryo transfer with a full bladder immediately before the real transfer for in-vitro fertilisation treatment: the Birmingham experience of 113 cases. *Hum Reprod* 1995; 10:1715–8.

7. Sallam HN. Embryo transfer: factors involved in optimizing the success. *Curr Opin Obstet Gynecol* 2005; 17:289–98.

8. Henne MB, Milki AA. Uterine position at real embryo transfer compared with mock embryo transfer. *Hum Reprod* 2004; 19: 570–2.

9. Yoldemir T, Erenus M. Does the timing of mock embryo transfer trial improve implantation in intracytoplasmic sperm injection cycles? *Gynecol Endocrinol* 2011; 27:396–400.

10. Katariya KO, Bates GW, Robinson RD, Arthur NJ, Propst AM. Does the timing of mock embryo transfer affect in vitro fertilization implantation and pregnancy rates? *Fertil Steril* 2007; 88:1462–4.

11. Sharif K, Afnan M, Lenton W. Mock embryo transfer with a full bladder immediately before the real transfer for in-vitro fertilization treatment: the Birmingham experience of 113 cases. *Hum Reprod* 1995; 10:1715–8.

12. Torre A, Scheffer JB, Schönauer LM, Frydman N, Fanchin R. Mock embryo transfer does not affect uterine contractility. *Fertil Steril* 2010; 93:1343–6.

13. Allahbadia GN, Kadam KS, Gandhi GN, Mhatre YP, Arora S. Pregnancy outcomes in IVF cycles with trial embryo transfer done 1 month prior to the cycle versus those done on the day of ET. *Fertil Steril* 2005; 84:S362.

14. Knutzen V, Stratton CJ, Sher G et al. Mock embryo transfer in early luteal phase, the cycle before in vitro fertilization and embryo transfer: a descriptive study. *Fertil Steril* 1992; 57:156–62.

15. Lesny P, Killick SR, Tetlow RL, Robinson J, Maguiness SD. Uterine junctional zone contractions during assisted reproduction cycles. *Hum Reprod Update* 1998; 4:440–5.

16. Zhu L, Xiao L, Che HS, Li YP, Liao JT. Uterine peristalsis exerts control over fluid migration after mock embryo transfer. *Hum Reprod* 2014; 29:279–85.

17. Eytan O, Elad D, Zaretsky U, Jaffa AJ. A glance into the uterus during in vitro simulation of embryo transfer. *Hum Reprod* 2004; 19:562–9.

18. Lesny P, Killick SR, Robinson J, Raven G, Maguiness SD. Junctional zone contractions and embryo transfer: is it safe to use a tenaculum? *Hum Reprod* 1999; 14: 2367–70.

19. Egbase PE, Al-Sharhan M, Grudzinskas JG. Influence of position and length of uterus on implantation and clinical pregnancy rates in IVF and embryo transfer treatment cycles. *Hum Reprod* 2000; 15:1943–6.

20. Karande VC, Morris R, Chapman C, Rinehart J, Gleicher N. Impact of the physician factor on pregnancy rates in a large assisted reproductive technology program: do too many cooks spoil the broth? *Fertil Steril* 1999; 71:1001–9.

21. Papageorgiou TC, Hearns-Stokes RM, Leondires MP et al. Training of providers in embryo transfer: what is the minimum number of transfers required for proficiency? *Hum Reprod* 2001; 16:1415–9.

22. Bishop L, Brezina PR, Segars J. Training in embryo transfer: how should it be done? *Fertil Steril* 2013; 100:351.

23. Shah DK, Missmer SA, Correia KF, Racowsky C, Ginsburg E. Efficacy of intrauterine inseminations as a training modality for performing embryo transfer in reproductive endocrinology and infertility fellowship programs. *Fertil Steril* 2013; 100:386–91.

24. Sinclair L, Morgan C, Lashen H, Afnan M, Sharif K. Nurses performing embryo transfer: the development and results of the Birmingham experience. *Hum Reprod* 1998; 3:699–702.

25. Neithardt AB, Segars JH, Hennessy S, James AN, McKeeby JL. Embryo after loading: a refinement in embryo transfer technique that may increase clinical pregnancy. *Fertil Steril* 2005; 83:710–4.

Chapter 12

Does Catheter Type Influence Endometrial Implantation Success?

Tia Hunjan, Shirin Khanjani and Stuart Lavery

12.1 Introduction

Ever since the first successful in vitro fertilisation (IVF) pregnancy in 1978, various aspects of this technology have been refined, leading to an increase in success rates. However, embryo transfer technique has remained relatively unchanged over time. Arguably, embryo transfer is a crucial step in the process of IVF, as whilst approximately 80 per cent of patients undergoing the journey reach this stage, a relatively small proportion actually achieves a pregnancy [1].

Compared with other aspects of IVF such as ovarian stimulation protocols and embryo culture, little attention has been given to the embryo transfer technique in the literature. This is perhaps due to the apparent simplicity of the task. However, data have shown that pregnancy rates vary between individuals performing the embryo transfer [13, 2], emphasising the importance of the technique. Thus, the process of embryo transfer has come under increasing scrutiny in recent years.

A number of factors may affect the likelihood of success of an embryo transfer, such as the operator's experience, presence of blood and mucus on the transfer catheter, the use of a trial (mock) transfer, ultrasound guidance, catheter-loading technique and catheter type [3].

The remainder of this chapter will focus on the influence of catheter type on implantation success.

12.2 Catheter Types

The ideal embryo transfer catheter possesses the following qualities:

  i. Able to navigate through the cervix into the uterine cavity
 ii. Minimises trauma to the cervix and endometrium
iii. Protects the embryo(s) and is able to deposit them in the appropriate location [4].

A traumatic embryo transfer is associated with a lower pregnancy rate due to the stimulation of uterine contractions, following trauma to the cervix or endometrium, which may cause expulsion of the embryo. The use of a tenaculum to grasp the cervix, or cervical dilators, may also cause uterine contractions and hence reduce success rates [4].

Various types of embryo transfer catheter are commercially available, mainly manufactured with non-toxic plastic materials or metal. Transfer catheters are broadly divided into two groups: soft and firm. There are further variations in terms of length, diameter of the lumen, location of the distal port (side or end-loading) and presence of an introducing cannula.

Soft catheters are thought to navigate the cervical canal and endometrial cavity with greater ease atraumatically, hence minimising the risk of trauma and of blood or mucus blocking the transfer tip. The main disadvantage of soft catheters is that they may be more difficult to insert, particularly with a very anteverted or anteflexed uterus; hence, firm catheters may be preferred in some circumstances.

12.2.1 Trauma Caused by Catheters

A small prospective descriptive study of 23 patients [6] was carried out to visualise possible trauma to the endocervix and endometrium, caused by the Tom Cat®, Frydman®'s catheter, Frydman®'s set and Wallace®'s embryo transfer catheters. They described various injuries

Table 12.1 The following table details some of the different embryo transfer catheters. Adapted from [5]

	Brand name	Detail
Soft	Frydman®	23 cm long inner polyurethrane catheter with external diameter 1.53 mm with open end.
	Edwards-Wallace®	Firm outer Teflon introducer. 18–23 cm long inner silicon catheter with external diameter 1.6 mm and open end.
	Cook® Soft-Pass	Two parts – inner and outer sheath. Length 27 cm. Tip contains stainless steel band within a polyethylene sheath to enable its visualisation during transabdominal ultrasound.
	Cook® Soft-Trans	Single lumen cannula. 12.5 cm firm proximal part and 4 cm soft distal part. Polyurethrane material.
	Cook® Sydney IVF®	Double lumen catheter set. Outer (guiding) catheter 19 cm long with angled distal end. Inner (transfer) catheter 23 cm long.
	Gynetics® Delphin	Single lumen catheter set, 21 cm. Combination of soft, flexible intra-uterine catheter and firm cervix catheter.
Firm	Erlangen®	Introducing metal cannula and insertion catheter. External diameter 2 mm, olive-shaped tip with diameter 3 mm. 25 cm length.
	Tom Cat®	Polyethylene. 11.5 mm long. External tip diameter 1 mm, internal 0.3 mm. Fits onto 1 ml syringe.
	Tight Difficult Transfer (TDT) ® Rochford Medical	Single lumen 18 cm long polyethylene/polypropylene cannula with partly polyethylene, partly metal transfer catheter. Equipped with malleable metal obturator allowing bending through cervical canal.
	Rocket® Embryon	18 cm length. Inner transfer catheter polyurethrane and outer sheath white polythene.
	Gynetics® Emtrac-A	Single lumen catheter set. 21 cm length. Flexible intra-uterine catheter and solid cervix catheter.

with each catheter and discovered that even with apparently 'easy' transfers trauma could be caused and that, overall, the Wallace® catheter appeared to be the least traumatic, in many cases causing no injury at all. However, even with this catheter, care must be taken not to pass the outer sheath through the internal os unless absolutely necessary, as this can cause significant damage and its diameter may initiate uterine contractions, which may affect implantation rates (IRs).

12.3 Outcomes with Different Catheter Types

Most early research consisted of large retrospective studies, generally showing increased success rates with 'softer' catheters [7]. However, one must bear in mind that technically difficult transfers may warrant the use of a hard catheter; hence, the lower pregnancy rate may be attributable to the inherent difficulties in the transfer process, rather than the catheter itself.

Results were, however, conflicting, with some randomised trial studies showing no difference in outcome between firm and soft catheters. Ghazzawi and colleagues [8] randomised 320 patients to the use of an Erlangen® metal catheter versus a Wallace® catheter. There was reduced need for the use of uterine sounding in the Erlangen® group and a significant increase in mucus blocking the tip of the Wallace® catheter and retained embryos after transfer. The overall increased pregnancy rate seen in the Erlangen® group did not reach clinical significance.

Following conflicting results from small underpowered studies, two meta-analyses were performed comparing firm and soft catheters. Firstly, Abou-Setta and colleagues [5] identified 23 randomised controlled trials (RCTs) evaluating different embryo transfer catheter types in both IVF and intra-cytoplasmic sperm injection (ICSI) cycles. Ten studies compared firm versus soft catheters, comprising a total of 4,141 embryo transfers. Primary outcome measures included IR, clinical pregnancy rate (CPR) and take-home baby rate. Notably, only two studies performed a sample size calculation.

Data for implantation were only available for two studies [9, 10], which failed to show a statistically significant difference in IR between soft (103/573) and firm (60/130) catheter use when analysed using a random effects model. Because of the heterogeneity, the results were reanalysed without the moderate quality study [8], which demonstrated increased IR rates with soft catheters ($p=0.001$).

Similarly, CPR was found to be higher for soft catheters when data were analysed using both the fixed and random effects models, adjusting for heterogeneity. The meta-analysis is shown in Figure 12.1.

With regard to secondary outcome measures, there was an increase in catheter failure with soft catheters, but this did not reach statistical significance. There was also an increased incidence in traumatic events using the soft versus firm catheters. Soft catheters were also associated with an increased need for use of a tenaculum, sounding and cervical dilatation during embryo transfer. Additionally, softer catheters were associated with a significantly increased risk of blood and mucus on the tip of the catheter and also retained embryos.

A subsequent review and meta-analysis [7] identified seven prospective trials comparing soft with hard catheters. The main outcome measure was CPR per embryo transfer. The studies were deemed to be relatively homogenous with minimal publication bias. Three thousand and sixty-three embryo transfers were examined in total demonstrating an increased chance of clinical pregnancy with soft catheters (Figure 12.2).

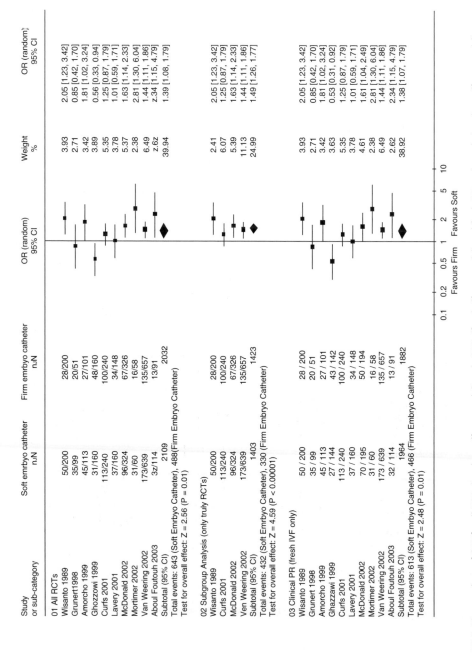

Figure 12.1 Meta-analysis of CPR for all RCTs (random effects model), truly RCTs (fixed effects model) and fresh IVF cycles only (random effects model)

Source: Abou-Setta, *Hum Reprod.* 2005.

Relative risk for clinical pregnancy per embryo transfer in trials comparing the TDT catheter with both hard and soft embryo transfer catheters (over unity in favor of TDT catheters).

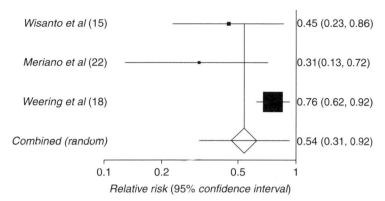

Relative risk meta-analysis plot (random effects)

Wisanto et al (15)	0.45 (0.23, 0.86)
Meriano et al (22)	0.31(0.13, 0.72)
Weering et al (18)	0.76 (0.62, 0.92)
Combined (random)	0.54 (0.31, 0.92)

Relative risk (95% confidence interval)

Figure 12.2 Buckett. Meta-analysis of ET catheters
Source: Fertil Steril 2006.

The TDT® hard catheter was associated with a reduced CPR when compared to the Frydman® hard catheter, the Wallace® soft catheter, the Tomcat® hard catheter and the Cook® soft catheter (Figure 12.3). It is important to note that a random effects model was used here due to increased statistical heterogeneity. Within the category of soft catheters, the Cook® and Wallace® catheters were compared in six relatively homogenous prospective trials, with reported minimal publication bias. Examination of 1277 embryo transfers revealed no significant difference in CPR between the two soft catheters (Figure 12.1). On the contrary, the earlier RCT by Wisanto and colleagues [11], which was not included in this review, reported a significantly higher CPR with the Frydman® (32.3 per cent) versus Wallace® (19.2 per cent) and TDT ® (9.2 per cent) catheter. A possible theory for the discrepancies includes differences in embryo transfer operator with different catheters. Although the pregnancy rates did not significantly differ between operators, pregnancy rates for each operator with each catheter type were not studied, and although randomisation occurred, it is possible that more operators with better experience with the Frydman® catheter and fewer operators with better experience with the Wallace® catheter performed embryo transfers in this study, leading to the impression of a higher CPR with the Frydman® catheter. Overall, the review concluded that softer catheters led to a more favourable outcome. Although no individual RCT had sufficient power to detect a 5 per cent difference in CPR with 80 per cent power (which would require a sample size of 2,500, assuming a CPR of 25 per cent and a significance level of 0.05 per cent), the combination of studies (3,063 embryo transfers) has a power of 97 per cent to detect a difference of 4.8 per cent in CPR. The authors comment on the possible impact of publication and selection bias in their outcome, although their funnel plot suggested this was unlikely. Additionally, it is important to note that the Frydman® catheter was categorised as soft in the 2005 meta-analysis and firm in Buckett's systematic review.

The higher CPR with softer catheters may be attributable to less damage to the endometrium and a resultant reduction in uterine contractions, which may affect implantation and pregnancy rates.

Relative risk for clinical pregnancy per embryo transfer in trials comparing soft with hard embryo transfer catheters (over unity in favor of soft catheters).

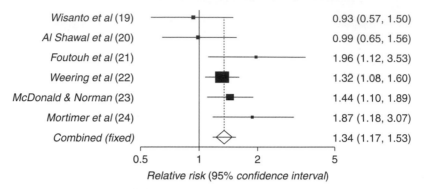

Relative risk meta-analysis plot (fixed effects)

Wisanto et al (19)	0.93 (0.57, 1.50)
Al Shawal et al (20)	0.99 (0.65, 1.56)
Foutouh et al (21)	1.96 (1.12, 3.53)
Weering et al (22)	1.32 (1.08, 1.60)
McDonald & Norman (23)	1.44 (1.10, 1.89)
Mortimer et al (24)	1.87 (1.18, 3.07)
Combined (fixed)	1.34 (1.17, 1.53)

Relative risk (95% confidence interval)

Figure 12.3 Buckett. Meta-analysis of ET catheters
Source: Fertil Steril 2006.

12.3.1 Degree of Difficulty

The degree of difficulty of embryo transfer, which can be affected by catheter type, is known to be an independent factor influencing success rates. A 2013 review [12] demonstrated a reduction in CPR with 'difficult transfers'. Difficult transfers were defined both subjectively and by the need for additional manoeuvres such as manipulation of the embryo transfer catheter, or use of a tenaculum or stylet. However, this review did not control for the effect of different catheter types, the use of ultrasound guidance, mock transfers or experience of the operator, and acknowledged that further systematic reviews on each of these aspects are warranted.

12.3.2 Operator Dependence

An interesting paper by Yao and colleagues [13] critiqued the two major systematic reviews on the topic of embryo transfer catheter type for their inclusion of many underpowered prospective trials analysed in a univariate manner (comparing CPR with catheter type). Although the meta-analysis itself is thought to somewhat compensate for the lack of power of individual trials, this would inevitably affect the overall value. Additionally, this paper comments on confusion regarding classification of some of the catheters as firm or soft in the reviews.

Their study compared the Cook® K-SOFT-5100 catheter with the Frydman® catheter in a large randomised trial, performing complex statistical analyses to determine the cause for previous inconsistencies in the literature. One thousand four hundred and forty-six embryo transfers were analysed in women undergoing both IVF and ICSI treatments. Primary analysis revealed no significant difference in CPR between the two catheters, which was confirmed on secondary analysis, adjusting for many baseline and cycle characteristics. Most interestingly, tertiary analysis revealed a significant interaction between the transfer catheter and operator ($p=0.0013$), suggesting this plays a significant role in success rates. Several of the previously published RCTs comparing catheter types tried to include operators with similar success rates to control for this effect, but do not comment on operator–catheter interactions specifically. Other RCTs have tried to eliminate the operator effect by using only one operator, although this of course limits the external validity of these RCTs. Only one previous RCT, comparing the TomCat® and Cook® catheter, controlled for operator in the same way as Yao and colleagues. They found greater inter-operator variability with the Cook® than the TomCat® catheter but the trial was underpowered to detect significant differences. Moving forward, a randomised trial sampling all embryo transfer operators is impractical and the only way to overcome this operator factor is by training.

12.4 Optimisation of Embryo Transfer Technique

12.4.1 Mock Transfer

The role of mock or dummy transfers in increasing the ease of embryo transfer is controversial [4]. It has been suggested that this process may assist in selecting the appropriate transfer catheter and provide information on navigating the cervical canal and endometrial cavity. For example, awareness of a severely anteverted uterus or a stenosed cervix requiring dilatation in advance may make the process of embryo transfer easier. This timing of the mock transfer, be it before ovarian stimulation, at oocyte collection or just before the embryo transfer, does not affect outcome.

12.4.2 Fixed Distance Technique

A retrospective review of 4,439 embryo transfers with an Edwards-Wallace® catheter in IVF and ICSI cycles by Van de Pas and colleagues [14] concluded that inter-operator variability can be reduced by consistently expelling embryos at 6 cm from the external os. They also found that this increased CPR. These findings were supported by a later prospective observational study of six physicians performing 977 embryo transfers with the fixed-distance technique with the Cook-K-soft 5000® catheter [15].

12.4.3 Ultrasound Guidance

Most studies included in the two systematic reviews on the topic of embryo transfer catheters did not perform embryo transfer under ultrasound guidance. Ultrasound guided embryo transfer (UGET) is thought to allow a more accurate and atraumatic deposition of embryos by allowing visualisation of the catheter tip. Disadvantages of UGET include the need for an additional operator, additional training, a longer procedure and possible disruption of the endometrium caused by manipulating the transfer catheter into vision.

A retrospective review [16] performed of 260 women undergoing a single embryo transfer concluded that the choice of catheter does not affect outcomes when the procedure is performed under ultrasound guidance. They used the Wallace® and Labotect® catheters and found no significant difference in CPR, implantation and ongoing pregnancy rates.

A recent Cochrane review [17] examined whether UGET improves pregnancy outcomes, compared with 'clinical touch'. Twenty-one RCTs were included involving 6,218 women. Type of transfer catheter used differed between groups. In the UGET cohort, 97 per cent of embryo transfers were carried out using the Cook® EchoTip, 1 per cent with Wallace® and 2 per cent with Rocket® catheters. In contrast, in the 'clinical touch' arm,

51 per cent used the Wallace® catheters, 47 per cent used the Rocket® catheters and only 2 per cent used the Cook® EchoTip. There was no significant difference in the live birth rate between groups. In studies where the same catheter was used in both groups (e.g. Frydman® and Labotect®), UGET was associated with a higher live birth rate.

A 2015 review [18] of the benefit of UGET compared with 'clinical touch' noted a similar finding of an increase in CPR, when using the same catheters and techniques. However, the review suggests that given the effect is not large, consideration should be given to the increased cost and training required for UGET.

12.5 Conclusion

In conclusion, there is inconsistent evidence in the literature regarding the role of catheter type in implantation success rates. Ultimately, an 'easy' and atraumatic embryo transfer is associated with the greatest chance of implantation. Systematic reviews have revealed an increased chance of success with soft catheters, although clearly certain circumstances warrant the use of a firmer catheter. Techniques to increase IRs include the use of a mock transfer and ultrasound guidance, and early studies have suggested that with UGET, catheter type has less influence on outcome. The use of ultrasound needs to be considered carefully, alongside the increased duration of the procedure, cost of a second operator and need for further training. Further large, RCTs are needed to confirm these findings.

References

1. Mansour, R. T. & Aboulghar, M. A. (2002). Optimizing the embryo transfer technique. *Human Reproduction, 17*(5), 1149–1153. doi:10.1093/humrep/17.5.1149

2. Hearns-Stokes, R. M., Miller, B. T., Scott, L. et al. (2000). Pregnancy rates after embryo transfer depend on the provider at embryo transfer. *Fertility and Sterility, 74*(1), 80–86. doi:10.1016/S0015-0282(00)00582-3

3. Derks, R. S., Farquhar, C., Mol, B. W. J., Buckingham, K., & Heineman, M. J. (2009). Techniques for preparation prior to embryo transfer. *Cochrane Database of Systematic Reviews*, (2). doi:10.1002/14651858.CD007682

4. Tiras, B., & Cenksoy, P. O. (2014). Practice of embryo transfer: Recommendations during and after. *Seminars in Reproductive Medicine, 32*: 291–296.

5. Abou-Setta, A. M., Al-Inany, H. G., Mansour, R. T., Serour, G. I., & Aboulghar, M. A. (2005). Soft versus firm embryo transfer catheters for assisted reproduction: A systematic review and meta-analysis. *Human Reproduction, 20*: 3114–3121.

6. Marconi, G., Vilela, Béllo J., Diradourián, Quintana R., & Sueldo C. (2003). Endometrial lesions caused by catheters used for embryo transfers: a preliminary report. *Fertil Steril, 80*: 363–367.

7. Buckett, W. (2006). A review and meta-analysis of prospective trials comparing different catheters used for embryo transfer. *Fertil Steril, 85*; 728–734.

8. Ghazzawi, I. M., Al-Hasani, S., Karaki, R., & Souso, S. (1999). Transfer technique and catheter choice influence the incidence of transcervical embryo expulsion and the outcome of IVF. *Hum Reprod, 14*: 677–682.

9. Grunert, G. M., Dunn, R. C., Valdes, C. T., Wunn, C. C., & Wunn, W. S. A. (1998). Comparison of Wallace, Frydman DY and Cook embryo transfer catheter for IVF: a prospective randomised study [abstract]. Annual meeting of the American Society of Reproductive Medicine. 1998. *Fertil Steril, 70*: S120.

10. Mortimer, S., Fluker, M., & Yuzpe, A. (2002). Effect of embryo transfer catheter on implantation rates [abstract]. 58th Annual General Meeting of the American Society for Reproductive Medicine. *Fertil Steril, 78*: S17–18.

11. Wisanto, A., Janssens, R., Camus, M., Devroey, P., & Van Steirteghem, A. C. (1989). Performance of different embryo transfer catheters in a human in vitro fertilization program. *Fertil Steril*, 52: 79–84.

12. Phillips, J. A, Martins, W. P, Nastri, C. O., & Raine-Fenning, N. J. (2013) Difficult embryo transfers or blood on catheter and assisted reproduction outcomes: a systematic review and meta-analysis. *Eur J Obstet Gynecol Reprod Biol*, 168: 121–128.

13. Yao, Z., Stijn, V., Van der Elst, J. et al. (2008). The efficacy of the embryo transfer catheter in IVF and ICSI is operator-dependent: a randomized clinical trial. *Hum Reprod*, 24: 880–887.

14. van de Pas, Weima S., Looman, C. W. N., Broekmans, F. J. M. (2003). The use of a fixed distance embryo transfer after IVF/ICSI equalizes the success rate among physicians. *Hum Reprod*, 18: 774–780.

15. van Weering, H. G., Schats, R., McDonnell, J., & Hompes, P.G. (2005). Ongoing pregnancy rates in in vitro fertilization are not dependent on the physician performing the embryo transfer. *Fertil Steril*, *83*: 316–320.

16. Aboulfotouh, I., Abou-Setta, A. M., Khattab, S., Mohsen, I. A., & Askalani, El-Din R. (2008). Firm versus soft embryo transfer catheters under ultrasound guidance: Does catheter choice really influence the pregnancy rates? *Fert Steril*, 89: 1261–1262.

17. Brown, J., Buckingham, K., Buckett, W., & Abou-Setta, A. M. (2016). Ultrasound versus "clinical touch" for catheter guidance during embryo transfer in women. *Cochrane Database of Systematic Reviews*, Issue 3. Art. No.: CD006107. DOI: 10.1002/14651858.CD006107.pub4.

18. Teixeira, D. M., Dassunção, L. A., & Vieira C. V, et al. (2015). Ultrasound-guidance during embryo transfer: a systematic review and meta analysis of randomized controlled trials. *Ultrasound Obstet Gynaecol*, 45: 139–148.

Chapter 13

Should All Embryos Be Transferred in Unstimulated Cycles?

Nikoletta Panagiotopoulou and Siladitya Bhattacharya

13.1 Introduction

Despite significant advances in assisted reproductive technology (ART), implantation and pregnancy rates have only risen slowly (20–40 per cent) over the last few years [1]. Embryo implantation involves a complex interaction between the embryo and the uterus, and, therefore, a receptive endometrium is critical for ART success.

Supraphysiological levels of oestradiol and progesterone observed after a hormonally stimulated in vitro fertilization (IVF) treatment cycle could affect endometrial development and perturb the interaction between embryo and endometrium [2]. Better understanding of cryobiology and the introduction of vitrification for embryo cryopreservation have meant that live birth rates following frozen embryo replacement are comparable with those observed after fresh embryo transfer [3]. This has allowed the ART community to seriously consider the potential benefits of a strategy where embryos are electively cryopreserved and transferred at a later date into an endometrium not exposed to supraphysiological levels of oestrogen, in order to improve ART success whilst minimizing risks. This approach is commonly referred to as 'freeze-all' or, more correctly, a 'freeze only' approach.

13.2 The Rationale for a Freeze-Only Approach

13.2.1 The Peri-Conception Milieu of Stimulated Cycles

Successful embryo implantation depends not only on embryo quality but also on endometrial receptivity and embryo-endometrial signalling which is influenced by the microenvironment of the uterine cavity. Therefore, understanding how the endometrium is affected in stimulation cycles is important in improving IVF outcomes.

During a menstrual cycle in normo-ovulatory women, the endometrium undergoes a number of sequential changes in preparation for the implantation of an embryo. These changes are driven by steroid hormones produced from the developing ovarian follicle, a process that ensures a degree of synchrony between endometrial development and oocyte maturity. Endometrial development involves proliferative changes in the first half of the cycle. After ovulation, secretory changes occur in the oestrogen-primed endometrium mainly through the action of progesterone produced by the luteinized follicle [4].

Results of genomic and immunohistological studies suggest that these physiological endometrial changes are altered during IVF cycles involving controlled ovarian hyperstimulation. Indeed, multi-follicular development, which is the aim of ovarian stimulation with exogenous hormones during an IVF cycle, exposes the endometrium to supraphysiological concentrations of oestrogen that accelerate endometrial proliferation. Stimulation-induced saturated steroid synthesizing capacity could subsequently lead to a shift towards earlier progesterone synthesis that induces premature endometrial secretory changes [5]. Women with high serum oestradiol concentrations during an IVF cycle have significantly more oocytes and higher levels of progesterone [6]. Moreover, patients with premature progesterone elevation have a reduced probability of clinical pregnancy in fresh embryo transfer cycles, but not in frozen/thawed or donor/recipient cycles [7].

In support of the clinical data, a number of basic science studies have shown dramatic differences between the normal cycling endometrium and the endometrium in women undergoing ovarian stimulation. Histological studies have shown that a pregnancy is unlikely to occur in IVF cycles involving gonadotropin-releasing hormone (GnRH) agonist or antagonist use, where endometrial advancement of three days or more is observed [8–10]. A comprehensive immune-histological study from Evans et al. has shown that ovarian stimulation could lead to a complex developmental asynchrony between the different endometrial cellular and structural compartments [11]. Indeed, this study demonstrated dramatic alterations in histological and immunochemical markers not only between endometrium from normal fertile women and women undergoing ovarian stimulation but also between endometrium from women who became pregnant after ovarian stimulation and those who did not. At the molecular level, alterations in both endometrial miRNA and mRNA expression are observed in women with elevated progesterone concentrations [12]. Transcriptomic studies have also revealed alterations in gene expression in the endometrium taken after ovarian stimulation, including elevation in DKK-I, which suggest the presence of an advanced endometrium [13]. Moreover, significant down-regulation of genes associated with implantation, including leukaemia inhibitory factor (LIF) and glycodelin, was observed in endometrial samples showing advanced maturation [14].

13.2.2 Clinical and Laboratory Advancements in Assisted Reproduction Technologies

Along with concerns about the non-physiologic peri-conception milieu of fresh IVF cycles, clinical and laboratory advancements in ART have contributed to a shift towards freeze-only policies.

A crucial step along the path towards a freeze-only approach was the introduction of vitrification where cells and tissues are exposed to high concentrations of cryoprotectants and rapid cooling rates. This combination aims to transform liquid to solid material without the formation of ice crystals, thus minimizing cell damage [15]. Available data show that the introduction of vitrification has led to enhanced embryo survival rates and improved clinical outcomes [16]. Vitrification has now been successfully employed not only to support a single-embryo transfer policy and optimize embryo utilization rates but also in the management of low [17] or hyper-responders [18], patients undergoing pre-implantation genetic testing (PGT) [19], as well in fertility preservation and donation programmes. However, cryopreservation, either through slow freezing or vitrification, could lead to morphological or developmental changes within the embryos. Indeed, vitrified-thawed blastocysts have shown increased spindle abnormalities when compared to fresh blastocysts [20]. Moreover, transcriptomic studies have revealed alterations in gene expression in vitrified-thawed embryos [21]. Cryopreservation and thawing is unlikely to improve embryo quality but may help to screen less competent embryos as embryos whose quality is already compromised are more likely to be adversely affected by cryopreservation and thawing [22].

The move towards safer IVF and avoidance of ovarian hyperstimulation syndrome (OHSS) are also contributing to the argument in support of a freeze-only approach. Human chorionic gonadotropin (hCG), which is used to induce the final follicular maturation instead of luteinizing hormone (LH) during IVF cycles, plays a crucial role in the development of OHSS. It has been shown that hCG stimulates vascular endothelial growth factor (VEGF) production in granulosa cells in vitro in a dose-dependent way and increases serum VEGF levels in vivo [23]. VEGF, which is a potent vasoactive peptide, is thought to play a pivotal role along with other inflammatory mediators in the pathogenesis of OHSS. Withholding hCG in treatment cycles with an excessive ovarian response to follicle-stimulating hormone (FSH) would, thus, eliminate the possibility of OHSS. As this is, however, an unpopular approach among clinicians and patients as it ultimately means cycle cancellation, antagonist protocols along with complementary measures, such as GnRH triggering, have been introduced. A meta-analysis has shown that GnRH agonist and antagonist protocols have similar live birth rates, with the latter being associated with a significantly lower incidence of OHSS [24]. However, GnRH triggering in the context of antagonist protocols has been associated with luteal phase defects that make fresh embryo transfer undesirable [25].

Moreover, the introduction of pre-implantation genetic testing (PGT) has made the freeze-all concept an attractive approach. In earlier stages, PGT was used to detect embryos with monogenic disorders (pre-implantation genetic diagnosis (PGD)). However, it has now expanded to include patients with no history of genetic disorders aiming to identify aneuploid embryos based on the commonly accepted premise that aneuploid embryos play a major role in failed implantation. Despite ongoing debate about its efficacy, pre-implantation genetic screening (PGS) is increasingly being used. From the technical point of view, PGT has evolved from biopsies of the polar body [26] to biopsies of cleavage-stage embryos [27] and, with advances in culture media formulations, to biopsies of blastocysts [28]. Advantages of blastocyst biopsy for PGT include reduced likelihood of embryo damage and mosaicism and increased DNA availability for testing at the expense of allowing for fresh embryo transfer, as time is needed for the results to become available. A freeze-only approach could thus help overcome time constraints associated with PGT in later embryo development stages.

13.3 Potential Benefits of a Freeze-Only and Delayed Embryo Transfer Approach

There are a number of arguments in support of a freeze-only approach with delayed embryo transfer in subsequent cycles. The concept of transferring embryos in a more physiological intra-uterine environment has strong biological plausibility as described earlier. Moreover, a move towards safer IVF with improved outcomes for mothers and offspring further supports this approach. Indeed, elective freezing of embryos and subsequent transfer in a future natural or medicated non-stimulation cycle can reduce the risk of OHSS or allow for PGT without compromising pregnancy rates.

A freeze-only approach might also show promise for addressing concerns about obstetric and perinatal outcomes after ART. Indeed, even though IVF is generally considered to be a safe medical intervention, pregnancies resulting from IVF are associated with poorer maternal and perinatal outcomes compared to spontaneous conceptions. Several studies have shown that children conceived after IVF are more likely to deliver preterm, have low birthweight or die during the perinatal period compared with those conceived without IVF treatment [29–31]. Among IVF pregnancies, obstetric and perinatal outcomes between fresh and frozen embryo transfers remain unclear. A systematic review and meta-analysis based on 11 observational studies showed that singleton pregnancies resulting from frozen embryo transfer were associated with lower obstetric and perinatal morbidity compared to those conceived following fresh embryo transfer [32]. The combined rate ratio (RR) of antepartum haemorrhage [0.67 (95 per cent confidence intervals (CI): 0.55, 0.81)], preterm birth [0.84 (0.78, 0.90)], low birthweight [0.69 (0.62, 0.76)] and perinatal mortality [0.68 (0.48, 0.96)] was lower after frozen embryo transfer. An observational study based on analysis of Nordic data [33], while endorsing some of these findings, has revealed that pregnancies resulting from frozen embryo transfer were at higher risk of post-term delivery [odds ratio 1.40 (95 per cent CI 1.27, 1.55)], large for gestational age [1.45 (1.27, 1.64)] or macrosomic [1.58 (1.39, 1.80)] and perinatal mortality [1.49 (1.07, 2.07)]. The above findings are in line with other population-based studies [34–36]. More recent evidence from another large observational study in the United Kingdom [37] has confirmed that singleton pregnancies resulting from frozen embryo transfer were at lower risk of low [RR 0.73 (99.5 per cent CI 0.66–0.80)] or very low birthweight [0.78 (0.63–0.96)], but at higher risk of high birthweight [1.64 (1.53–1.76)]. No difference in the incidence of preterm birth [0.96 (0.88–1.03)], very preterm birth [0.86 (0.70–1.05)] and congenital anomalies [0.86 (0.73–1.01)] was observed. It should be acknowledged that all these studies are observational and, therefore, their results could be confounded by differences in the characteristics of women undergoing fresh or frozen embryo transfer, differences in cryopreservation techniques or ART cycle characteristics.

A long-awaited randomized controlled trial (RCT) [38] comparing immediate transfer of cleavage-stage fresh embryos with delayed transfer of frozen embryos concluded that frozen embryo transfer in infertile women with polycystic ovarian syndrome resulted in a higher rate of live birth after the first embryo transfer cycle than did for fresh embryo transfer [RR 1.17 (95 per cent CI 1.05, 1.31)]. As expected, frozen embryo transfer was associated with lower incidence of OHSS in comparison to fresh embryo transfer [0.19 (0.10, 0.37)]. However, the incidence of pre-eclampsia was higher in the frozen embryo group than in the fresh embryo group [3.12 (1.26, 7.73)]. No significant between-group differences in terms of pregnancy and neonatal complications were seen, although there were two stillbirths and five neonatal deaths in the frozen embryo group and none in the fresh embryo group. Post hoc analysis showed higher birthweights in the frozen embryo group, a finding that is consistent with previous reports. The findings of this study provide reassurance that the transfer of both fresh and frozen embryos results in satisfactory live birth rates and that, therefore, vitrification of embryos is not detrimental in their ability to implant and result in the delivery of a live infant.

13.4　Potential Risks of a Freeze-Only and Delayed Embryo Transfer Approach

Before adopting a freeze-only approach with delayed embryo transfer in subsequent cycles, potential benefits should be carefully weighed against risks. Although current data suggest an improvement in most obstetric and perinatal outcomes after frozen embryo transfer, there are some perinatal outcomes that remain a source of concern. Indeed, as highlighted earlier, a number of studies have reported increased risk of large for gestational age and fetal macrosomia in offspring conceived following frozen embryo transfer, which may be linked to embryo freezing and thawing. Similarly, perinatal mortality appears to be higher in this group.

The clinical effectiveness and safety of a freeze-only approach with delayed embryo transfer in subsequent cycles has not yet been proven. Data on IVF success come from three RCTs on selected subgroups of women [38–40]. The studied population of these trials included normal or hyper-responders to ovarian stimulation, and, therefore, outcomes cannot be extrapolated to a wider population of women undergoing IVF. Only one of these RCTs [38] provided data on live birth rates while none of them provided data on cost-effectiveness or patient acceptability. Understanding patient preferences is important before adopting a freeze-only approach. Patients value reduced time to pregnancy, and, therefore, elective embryo freezing with delayed embryo transfer in subsequent cycles may appear counterintuitive. Moreover, an elective embryo freezing approach is associated with increased physical burden for patients who are required to undergo additional treatments involving the administration of hormones and close monitoring to ensure adequate endometrial preparation prior to embryo transfer. Similarly, clinicians or embryologists may be resistant to adopting an elective embryo freezing approach for fear of low post-thaw embryo survival rates. Finally, an elective embryo freezing approach is associated with higher incremental financial costs in comparison to a fresh embryo cycle of treatment.

13.5 Optimal Endometrial Preparation for Frozen Embryo Transfer

Several methods of endometrial preparation for frozen embryo transfer have been developed, including natural cycle protocols, where the endometrium is physiologically primed by sex steroids produced from the growing follicle, and artificial cycle protocols, where endometrial preparation is achieved with a combination of exogenous hormones. As pregnancy rates are closely dependent on the timely identification of ovulation and calculation of the likely subsequent period of optimal endometrial receptivity, a true natural cycle protocol demands close monitoring for timely identification of LH surge [41]. However, LH surge identification can be difficult due to significant intra- and inter-patient variation in timing of its occurrence as well as technical limitations of available detection kits. To overcome the disadvantages of LH monitoring, a modified natural cycle protocol can be employed where ovulation is triggered by hCG as soon as the dominant follicle reaches a sufficient size. Unexpected ovulation with subsequent cycle cancellation is one of the drawbacks of a natural cycle protocol.

In artificial cycle protocols, exogenous hormones are administered in order to simulate endocrine changes observed in a natural menstrual cycle. This includes the administration of oestradiol or gonadotropins in order to cause endometrial proliferation followed by administration of progesterone. GnRH agonist co-treatment maybe used to ensure pituitary down-regulation and prevent follicular growth and ovulation.

A number of groups have studied reproductive outcomes in frozen embryo transfer cycles using available endometrial preparation protocols. However, so far, available data have failed to show any differences between strategy, natural cycle versus a hormonally modulated cycle in ovulating women with a regular cycle. A systematic review of observational and RCTs [42] revealed no significant difference in live birth rates between natural and modified natural cycle [OR 0.82, 95 per cent CI (0.63, 1.08)], natural and artificial cycle using oestrogen and progesterone [1.23 (0.93, 1.62)], natural and artificial cycle supplemented with GnRH agonist [0.79 (0.52, 1.20)] or artificial cycle with or without GnRH agonist [0.79 (0.43, 1.43)]. More recent data from two more RCTs [43, 44] have failed to show a difference in reproductive outcomes observed among different endometrial preparation protocols used prior to frozen replacement transfer cycles. Since no significant difference in reproductive outcomes has been observed, the choice for either endometrial preparation strategy could be based on patient preferences and clinic logistics.

13.6 Indications for Freeze-Only Approach

As definitive evidence on the clinical and cost-effectiveness of a freeze-only approach with delayed embryo transfer in subsequent cycles is still lacking, recommendations need to be individualized. Elective freezing of all embryos offers advantages that outweigh disadvantages in selected groups of women undergoing IVF. Women who could benefit from a freeze-only approach are those at high risk of OHSS, such as women with polycystic ovarian syndrome, or predicted poor responders who want to adopt a strategy of oocyte or embryo 'batching'. Moreover, a freeze-only approach might be beneficial for women with an altered endocrine profile, such as prematurely elevated progesterone at the time of embryo transfer, or with inadequate uterine environment for embryo transfer, such as thin endometrium. Last but not least, a freeze-only approach may be a prerequisite for patients seeking pre-implantation genetic testing at blastocyst stage. However, the benefits of a freeze-only approach cannot yet be extrapolated to the general IVF population, and, therefore, elimination of fresh embryo transfer in IVF should not be generalized until definitive evidence from RCTs become available.

13.7 Conclusion

Advances in the field of cryobiology in ART have led to improved reproductive outcomes associated with the transfer of frozen embryos. Improved live birth rates along with concerns about adverse obstetric and perinatal outcomes in pregnancies after fresh embryo transfer have called into question the traditional strategy of fresh embryo transfer in stimulated IVF cycles. However, in the absence of definitive evidence on clinical and cost-effectiveness of a freeze-only approach, clinical decisions should be individualized according to predicted risk associated with fresh transfer, logistics and patient preferences.

References

1. Kupka MS, Ferraretti AP, de Mouzon J et al. Assisted reproductive technology in Europe, 2010: results generated from European registers by ESHREdagger. *Human Reproduction.* 2014;29:2099–113.

2. Evans J, Hannan NJ, Edgell TA et al. Fresh versus frozen embryo transfer: backing clinical decisions with scientific and clinical evidence. *Human Reproduction Update.* 2014;20:808–21.

3. Calhaz-Jorge C, de Geyter C, Kupka MS et al. Assisted reproductive technology in Europe, 2012: results generated from European registers by ESHRE. *Human Reproduction.* 2016;31:1638–52.

4. Noyes RW, Hertig AT, Rock J. Dating the endometrial biopsy. *American Journal of Obstetrics and Gynecology.* 1975;122:262–3.

5. Devroey P, Bourgain C, Macklon NS, Fauser BC. Reproductive biology and IVF: ovarian stimulation and endometrial

receptivity. *Trends Endocrinol Metab.* 2004;15:84–90.

6. Kyrou D, Kolibianakis EM, Venetis CA et al. How to improve the probability of pregnancy in poor responders undergoing in vitro fertilization: a systematic review and meta-analysis. *Fertility and Sterility.* 2009;91:749–66.

7. Venetis CA, Kolibianakis EM, Bosdou JK, Tarlatzis BC. Progesterone elevation and probability of pregnancy after IVF: a systematic review and meta-analysis of over 60 000 cycles. *Human Reproduction Update.* 2013;19:433–57.

8. Ubaldi F, Bourgain C, Tournaye H et al. Endometrial evaluation by aspiration biopsy on the day of oocyte retrieval in the embryo transfer cycles in patients with serum progesterone rise during the follicular phase. *Fertility and Sterility.* 1997;67:521–6.

9. Kolibianakis EM, Devroey P. The luteal phase after ovarian stimulation. *Reproductive Biomedicine Online.* 2002;5 Suppl 1:26–35.

10. Van Vaerenbergh I, Van Lommel L, Ghislain V et al. In GnRH antagonist/rec-FSH stimulated cycles, advanced endometrial maturation on the day of oocyte retrieval correlates with altered gene expression. *Human Reproduction.* 2009;24: 1085–91.

11. Evans J, Hannan NJ, Hincks C, Rombauts LJ, Salamonsen LA. Defective soil for a fertile seed? Altered endometrial development is detrimental to pregnancy success. *PloS one.* 2012;7e53098.

12. Labarta E, Martinez-Conejero JA, Alama P et al. Endometrial receptivity is affected in women with high circulating progesterone levels at the end of the follicular phase: a functional genomics analysis. *Human Reproduction.* 2011;26:1813–25.

13. Macklon NS, van der Gaast MH, Hamilton A, Fauser BC, Giudice LC. The impact of ovarian stimulation with recombinant FSH in combination with GnRH antagonist on the endometrial transcriptome in the window of implantation. *Reprod Sci.* 2008;15:357–65.

14. Horcajadas JA, Riesewijk A, Polman J et al. Effect of controlled ovarian hyperstimulation in IVF on endometrial gene expression profiles. *Molecular Human Reproduction.* 2005;11:195–205.

15. Luyet BJ, Hodapp EL. Revival of Frog's Spermatozoa Vitrified in Liquid Air. *Experimental Biology and Medicine.* 1938;39:433–34.

16. Rienzi L, Gracia C, Maggiulli R et al. Oocyte, embryo and blastocyst cryopreservation in ART: systematic review and meta-analysis comparing slow-freezing versus vitrification to produce evidence for the development of global guidance. *Human Reproduction Update.* 2017;23:139–55.

17. Cobo A, Garrido N, Crespo J, Jose R, Pellicer A. Accumulation of oocytes: a new strategy for managing low-responder patients. *Reproductive Biomedicine Online.* 2012;24:424–32.

18. Herrero L, Pareja S, Losada C et al. Avoiding the use of human chorionic gonadotropin combined with oocyte vitrification and GnRH agonist triggering versus coasting: a new strategy to avoid ovarian hyperstimulation syndrome. *Fertility and Sterility.* 2011;95:1137–40.

19. Chamayou S, Sicali M, Alecci C et al. The accumulation of vitrified oocytes is a strategy to increase the number of euploid available blastocysts for transfer after preimplantation genetic testing. *Journal of Assisted Reproduction and Genetics.* 2017. Epub 2017 January 9.

20. Chatzimeletiou K, Morrison EE, Panagiotidis Y et al. Cytoskeletal analysis of human blastocysts by confocal laser scanning microscopy following vitrification. *Human Reproduction.* 2012;27:106–13.

21. Tachataki M, Winston RM, Taylor DM. Quantitative RT-PCR reveals tuberous sclerosis gene, TSC2, mRNA degradation following cryopreservation in the human preimplantation embryo. *Molecular Human Reproduction.* 2003;9:593–601.

22. Van den Abbeel E, Camus M, Van Waesberghe L et al. Viability of partially

damaged human embryos after cryopreservation. *Human Reproduction.* 1997;12:2006–10.

23. Neulen J, Yan Z, Raczek S et al. Human chorionic gonadotropin-dependent expression of vascular endothelial growth factor/vascular permeability factor in human granulosa cells: importance in ovarian hyperstimulation syndrome. *The Journal of Clinical Endocrinology and Metabolism.* 1995;80:1967–71.

24. Al-Inany HG, Youssef MA, Ayeleke RO et al. Gonadotrophin-releasing hormone antagonists for assisted reproductive technology. *The Cochrane Database of Systematic Reviews.* 2016;4:CD001750.

25. Shapiro BS, Andersen CY. Major drawbacks and additional benefits of agonist trigger–not ovarian hyperstimulation syndrome related. *Fertility and Sterility.* 2015;103:874–78.

26. Munne S, Dailey T, Sultan KM, Grifo J, Cohen J. The use of first polar bodies for preimplantation diagnosis of aneuploidy. *Human Reproduction.* 1995;10:1014–20.

27. Hardy K, Handyside AH. Biopsy of cleavage stage human embryos and diagnosis of single gene defects by DNA amplification. *Arch Pathol Lab Med.* 1992;116:388–92.

28. McArthur SJ, Leigh D, Marshall JT, de Boer KA, Jansen RP. Pregnancies and live births after trophectoderm biopsy and preimplantation genetic testing of human blastocysts. *Fertility and Sterility.* 2005;84: 1628–36.

29. Helmerhorst FM, Perquin DA, Donker D, Keirse MJ. Perinatal outcome of singletons and twins after assisted conception: a systematic review of controlled studies. *BMJ.* 2004;328:261.

30. Henningsen AK, Pinborg A, Lidegaard O et al. Perinatal outcome of singleton siblings born after assisted reproductive technology and spontaneous conception: Danish national sibling-cohort study. *Fertility and Sterility.* 2011;95:959–63.

31. Pandey S, Shetty A, Hamilton M, Bhattacharya S, Maheshwari A. Obstetric and perinatal outcomes in singleton pregnancies resulting from IVF/ICSI: a systematic review and meta-analysis. *Human Reproduction Update.* 2012;18:485–503.

32. Maheshwari A, Pandey S, Shetty A, Hamilton M, Bhattacharya S. Obstetric and perinatal outcomes in singleton pregnancies resulting from the transfer of frozen thawed versus fresh embryos generated through in vitro fertilization treatment: a systematic review and meta-analysis. *Fertility and Sterility.* 2012;98:368–77 e1–9.

33. Wennerholm UB, Henningsen AK, Romundstad LB et al. Perinatal outcomes of children born after frozen-thawed embryo transfer: a Nordic cohort study from the CoNARTaS group. *Human Reproduction.* 2013;28:2545–53.

34. Sazonova A, Kallen K, Thurin-Kjellberg A, Wennerholm UB, Bergh C. Obstetric outcome in singletons after in vitro fertilization with cryopreserved/thawed embryos. *Human Reproduction.* 2012;27: 1343–50.

35. Roy TK, Bradley CK, Bowman MC, McArthur SJ. Single-embryo transfer of vitrified-warmed blastocysts yields equivalent live-birth rates and improved neonatal outcomes compared with fresh transfers. *Fertility and Sterility.* 2014;101: 1294–301.

36. Belva F, Bonduelle M, Roelants M, Verheyen G, Van Landuyt L. Neonatal health including congenital malformation risk of 1072 children born after vitrified embryo transfer. *Human Reproduction.* 2016;31:1610–20.

37. Maheshwari A, Raja EA, Bhattacharya S. Obstetric and perinatal outcomes after either fresh or thawed frozen embryo transfer: an analysis of 112,432 singleton pregnancies recorded in the Human Fertilisation and Embryology Authority anonymized dataset. *Fertility and Sterility.* 2016;106:1703–8.

38. Chen ZJ, Shi Y, Sun Y et al. Fresh versus Frozen Embryos for Infertility in the Polycystic Ovary Syndrome. *The New England journal of Medicine.* 2016;375: 523–33.

39. Shapiro BS, Daneshmand ST, Garner FC et al. Evidence of impaired endometrial receptivity after ovarian stimulation for in vitro fertilization: a prospective randomized trial comparing fresh and frozen-thawed embryo transfer in normal responders. *Fertility and Sterility*. 2011;96: 344–8.

40. Shapiro BS, Daneshmand ST, Garner FC et al. Evidence of impaired endometrial receptivity after ovarian stimulation for in vitro fertilization: a prospective randomized trial comparing fresh and frozen-thawed embryo transfers in high responders. *Fertility and Sterility*. 2011;96: 516–18.

41. Harper MJ. The implantation window. *Baillieres Clin Obstet Gynaecol*. 1992;6: 351–71.

42. Groenewoud ER, Cantineau AE, Kollen BJ, Macklon NS, Cohlen BJ. What is the optimal means of preparing the endometrium in frozen-thawed embryo transfer cycles? A systematic review and meta-analysis. *Human Reproduction Update*. 2017;23:255–61

43. Peeraer K, Couck I, Debrock S et al. Frozen-thawed embryo transfer in a natural or mildly hormonally stimulated cycle in women with regular ovulatory cycles: a RCT. *Human Reproduction*. 2015;30:2552–62.

44. Groenewoud ER, Cohlen BJ, Al-Oraiby A et al. A randomized controlled, non-inferiority trial of modified natural versus artificial cycle for cryo-thawed embryo transfer. *Human Reproduction*. 2016;31:1483–92.

Rest after Embryo Transfer Is Unhelpful

Giuseppe Botta and Gedis Grudzinskas

14.1 Introduction

Attitudes towards physical activity and other aspects of our daily life form part of the in vitro fertilisation (IVF) care strategies. Assisted reproduction technology (ART) centres and 'gurus', also well intentioned, offer guidance which is rarely evidence-based regarding diet, levels of physical activity and work-related matters. There is now a strengthening database regarding physical activity after embryo transfer (ET) from which information can be derived to reduce the avoidable stress many couples endure at this time, minimally medicalising their lives without threatening the best outcome of their IVF treatment. The effect of gravity when standing after ET, position of the uterus during and after ET, levels of physical activity immediately after the ET procedure and in the following 24 hours, even 14 days, are the confounding variables which have been scrutinised. There is also evidence that exercise is beneficial, leaving couples potentially confused as to how to deal with conflicting information implying the benefits of inactivity after ET, from ART centres and other authoritative sources, as well as cleverly worded social network sites. The former are expected to be evidence-based and, as such, should be persuasive, but are not; the latter, which grow in number almost daily, reflect the professionals' poor communication skills or lack of interest, leaving couples vulnerable to commercial interests of the internet wilderness.

'What will happen when I stand up?' This is the question often asked, or worse not asked, by women undergoing either intra-uterine insemination or ET. Formerly, in the absence of evidence, the tendency had been to advise women to remain horizontal for a short period or for longer intervals to full bed rest for 24 hours. The new reality is that bed rest may have a negative effect.

Is there sufficient anecdotal evidence that remaining horizontal immediately after ET for some time may be helpful, a matter which to some unjustifiably fuels anxiety of women and their husbands/partners? As there is no evidence to support this and there is evidence to the contrary, we should actively ensure that these issues are addressed with the best information now available.

This short review updates the literature on whether rest after ET will improve live birth rates, once again reaching the conclusion that there is no evidence that it is helpful and in fact indicates that it is unhelpful. Is there any reason why we should not, in all circumstances, advise all our patients immediately after ET to rise and resume their normal daily activities, subject to having recovered from their oocyte retrieval surgery a few days previously?

14.2 Bed Rest and Reduced Physical Activity after Embryo Transfer: The Early Years of IVF

Historically, bed rest following ET was advised given the conservative medical approach at the time that bed rest facilitates the recovery process, notably from the then more invasive techniques (laparoscopic or transurethral/vesical) of oocyte retrieval, and by inference facilitate implantation. Such guidance was likely to have been meticulously followed, given the deferential attitude towards professional advice at that time and the pioneering nature of this fertility treatment. Given the less invasive nature of procedures and the wealth of experience of ET in women who have not had oocyte collection recently (frozen-thawed embryo transfer, FET) as well as women whose embryos have been derived using donor oocytes, patients and doctors alike began to reconsider traditional practice of restricted activities following ET. Understandably, it is not easy for someone who is and feels well to comply with advice to remain in bed or horizontal for prolonged periods of time unless this can be justified. Women and ART professionals began to question the need for such a hard-line position on restriction of almost all activity after ET for at least a day. Well intentioned, though this approach may have been, it soon began to be challenged as more women became pregnant following ET not having been on full bed rest because they would not or simply could not afford to be immobilised either at home or in a hospital bed. Thus, in accord with many other changes in medical and surgical practice, not just in ART, the relevance of such conservative approaches began to be questioned and to some degree subjected to scientific scrutiny.

14.3 The Naples Study

We compared 20 minutes of bed rest with 24 hours bed rest following ET and showed that rest for 24 hours following ET is not associated with a better outcome than when compared to bed rest for 20 minutes [1] We stated: 'Women, a few minutes after embryo transfer, can stand, empty their bladder and return home with no apparent risk to the process of implantation. No restriction of the routine activity of the patients need be advised after the transfer. This observation has some important economic implications: a short bed rest following embryo transfer avoids an extra day of recovery in the clinic and its related costs. Moreover, the early return of the patient to her daily activities allows an immediate return to work with no loss in productivity.'

As one of the earliest RCTs on this subject challenging the received wisdom, it was difficult to assess quite what impact, if any, our report had or would have. One may speculate that our conclusion provided reassurance for some women who, of necessity, needed to be immediately ambulant, or to being ignored by the ART professionals at large. Nevertheless, some women instinctively feel that rest is helpful, for peace of mind, if nothing else. Subsequent studies, typically observational, confirmed our findings, and as the efficiency of ART improved, most centres reporting two- to threefold increases in live birth rates to those seen in the 1980s, more robust study designs were used to address the benefits or not of immobilisation/bed rest immediately after ET and subsequently.

14.4 The Netherlands Study, Cochrane Database Systematic Review

Data from later robust studies, such as that of Lambers and colleagues, have been in accord, as well as recommending that bed rest after ET is useless [2].

Abou-Setta and colleagues [3] on behalf of the Cochrane Library performed screening and selection of 2,436 possible trial citations independently by two review authors. Four prospective, truly randomised controlled trials (RCTs) met the inclusion criteria. The trials compared two competing post-ET interventions, or an intervention versus no treatment, in women undergoing IVF and ICSI. With respect to bed rest after ET, the primary outcome, live birth rate, was not reported in any of the included trials and the ongoing pregnancy rate was only available for one trial that compared immediate ambulation with 30-minute bed rest, with no evidence of an effect with bed rest (OR 1.00; 95 per cent CI 0.54–1.85). Secondary outcomes were sporadically reported with the exception of clinical pregnancy rate, which was reported in all of the included trials. There was no significant difference between less bed rest and more rest (OR 1.13; 95 per cent CI 0.77–1.67).

Gaikwad and colleagues [4] recruited recipients of embryos derived from good prognosis oocyte donors, correcting for confounding variables which potentially compromised the conclusions from all earlier studies. Their observation that the live birth rate was statistically significantly higher in the non-rest group (56.7 per cent vs. 41.6 per cent: p=0.02) has provided a firm evidence on which current recommendations to patients should be based.

14.5 Taking the Embryo for a Walk?

Kucuk and colleagues [5] added novel evidence of the beneficial effects of moderate levels of exercise for women undergoing ART, reporting substantially higher implantation and live birth rates than if there was less exercise. Given that ART involves minor surgery for the oocyte retrieval, it is not a surprise that women do not have high levels of activity, but their data indicate that immobilisation or reduced physical activity should not be advised. It is notable that none of the women undergoing ART had a high level of activity, so an enquiry about physical activity and reinforcing/advising women to maintain their normal moderate level of activity makes complete sense. As advice on the woman's usual level of physical activity after ET is not an intervention, whether the better outcomes result from exercise-induced benefits acting directly on the implantation process or via complex neuroendocrine pathways is of secondary relevance, if any.

14.6 UK National Institute of Clinical Excellence (NICE) Guidelines (2017)

The UK National Institute of Clinical Excellence (NICE) in 2017 issued NICE Clinical Guidelines 011 for Fertility [6], which included the following recommendation:

'Women should be informed that bed rest of more than 20 minutes' duration following embryo transfer does not improve the outcome of IVF treatment', citing Grade A as the strength of evidence for this recommendation, being at least one RCT.

14.7 American Society of Reproductive Medicine (2017)

The American Society of Reproductive Medicine (ASRM) standard embryo transfer protocol [7] states: 'Step 12: the patient gets up from the transfer table and leaves the room immediately, without being provided routinely any period of bed rest first (Systematic Review and Common Practice). The guideline states that there is good evidence not to recommend bed rest after ET (Grade A) (ASRM standard embryo transfer protocol template: a committee opinion).

14.8 Conclusion

There is now persuasive data to advise all our patients immediately after ET to rise and resume their normal daily activities, subject to having recovered from their oocyte retrieval surgery a few days previously. In the following days, although seemingly counter–intuitive, as taking (the embryo for) regular walks or other forms of moderate exercise will lead to a higher chance of live birth, women should be encouraged to do so.

References

[1] Botta G, Grudzinskas G. Is a prolonged bed rest following embryo transfer useful? *Human Reproduction* 1997;12:2489–2492.

[2] Lambers MJ, Lambalk CB, Schats R, Hompes PG. Ultrasonographic evidence that bed rest after embryo transfer is useless. *Gynecol Obstet Invest.* 2009;68:122–126.

[3] Abou-Setta AM, D'Angelo A, Sallam HN, Hart RJ, Al-Inany HG. Post-embryo transfer interventions for in vitro fertilization and intracytoplasmic sperm injection patients. *Cochrane Database Syst Rev.* 2009 October 7; (4):CD006567.

[4] Gaikwad S, Garrido N, Cobo A, Pellicer A, Remohi J. Bed rest after embryo transfer negatively affects in-vitro fertilization: a randomized controlled clinical trial. *Fertility and Sterility* 2013;100:729–735.

[5] Kucuk M, Doymaz F, Urman B. Effect of energy expenditure and physical activity on the outcomes of assisted reproduction treatment. *RBMOnline* 2010;20:274–279.

[6] The UK National Institute of Clinical Excellence (NICE). NICE *Clinical Guidelines 011 for Fertility* 2004; 112–114.

[7] ASRM standard embryo transfer protocol template: a committee opinion. Practice Committee of American Society of Reproductive Medicine. *Fertility and Sterility* 2017;107:879–900.

Chapter 15

Ectopic Pregnancies: Why Do They Happen?

Rohan Chodankar and Andrew Horne

15.1 Introduction

Ectopic pregnancies represent 1–2 per cent of all pregnancies and are responsible for significant maternal morbidity and mortality [1, 2]. In the United Kingdom, the rate of ectopic pregnancy is 11 per 1000 pregnancies, with a maternal mortality of 0.2 per 1000 estimated ectopic pregnancies. An ectopic pregnancy is defined as a pregnancy implanted outside the normal uterine cavity, and over 98 per cent implant in the Fallopian tube.

In this chapter, we present the current evidence explaining the aetiology of the tubal ectopic pregnancy (Table 15.1). However, our current understanding of why tubal ectopic pregnancies occur is limited by a lack of good animal models (animals are more likely to develop abdominal rather than tubal ectopic pregnancies [3]) and relies heavily on descriptive ex-vivo human data.

Table 15.1 Summary of maternal factors in the aetiology of tubal ectopic pregnancy

Factor	Expression in the Fallopian tube of women with tubal ectopic pregnancy	Probable effect
Interstitial cells of Cajal (ICC)	Reduced	Reduced tubal motility
Nitric oxide (NO)	Increased	Reduced tubal motility
Prokinecticin receptors (PROKRs)	Reduced	Reduced tubal motility
Endocannabinoid receptor (CB1)	Reduced	Reduced tubal motility
Mucin 1 (MUC1)	Reduced	More receptive tubal microenvironment
Interleukin 8 (IL-8)	Increased	Tubal damage leading to a more receptive tubal microenvironment
Activins	Increased	Reduced tubal motility. More receptive tubal microenvironment

There are several recognised risk factors associated with the development of a tubal ectopic pregnancy [2, 4–6].

- Cigarette smoking
- Pelvic *Chlamydia trachomatis (C. trachomatis)* infection
- *Neisseria gonorrhoea* infection
- Previous tubal surgery
- In vitro fertilisation (IVF)

Proposed mechanisms of how these risk factors may cause an ectopic pregnancy include the following:

1. Retention of the embryo in the Fallopian tube due to impaired tubal-embryo transport
2. Changes in the tubal micro-environment
3. A combination of the above

15.2 Role of the Tubal Smooth Muscle and Epithelium

Effective tubal-embryo transport is regulated by smooth muscle contractility and ciliary beat activity within the Fallopian tube [7, 8].

15.2.1 Ciliary Beat Activity

The mucosa of the Fallopian tube is arranged as folds and consists of a single layer of epithelium (columnar or cuboidal) with two distinct cell types, secretory and ciliated. The ciliated cells are predominantly found at the apex of the mucosal folds.

Ciliary beat frequency increases during the mid-luteal phase, suggesting a strong progesterone influence. In addition to sex steroid hormones, prostaglandins and other factors from the ovarian follicle fluid are also thought to regulate ciliary activity [8–10]. Reduced numbers of ciliated cells are found in Fallopian tubes of women who have had an ectopic pregnancy and in women following tubal surgery who subsequently go on to develop one [11]. De-ciliation associated with an up-regulation of tumour necrosis factor-alpha (TNF-α) is seen to occur after tubal infection with *Neisseria gonorrhoea* [12]. Animal studies have demonstrated reduced ciliary beat frequency after exposure to cigarette smoke [13].

15.2.2 Smooth Muscle Contractility

The factors that regulate tubal smooth muscle contractility include the following:

- Interstitial cells of Cajal (ICCs)
- Nitric oxide (NO)
- Prokinecticins (PROK)
- Endocannabinoids
- Adrenergic neurons

15.2.3 Interstitial Cells of Cajal [14–16]

ICCs are pacemaker cells expressed in the human Fallopian tube and are thought to regulate smooth muscle contractility. They are (dominantly) resident in the Fallopian tube ampullary region, in the lamina propria, immediately under the tubal epithelium and in between smooth muscle fibres.

These cells express the progesterone receptor and are thought to thereby mediate progesterone control of tubal motility. Animal studies reveal that *C. trachomatis* infection of the Fallopian tube is associated with a loss of ICCs either due to apoptosis or reduced proliferation and up-regulation of inducible nitric oxide synthase (iNOS) with resultant disruption of the pacemaker activity and smooth muscle contractility regulated by the ICCs.

15.2.4 Nitric Oxide

NO has been shown to induce relaxation of tubal smooth muscle [17]. NO is synthesised from L-arginine by nitric oxide synthase (NOS). The levels of NOS expression are found to be higher in the Fallopian tubes of women with past tubal ectopic pregnancies [18]. Animal studies using mice infected with *C. muridarum* have shown an increased NOS expression [14], potentially explaining the correlation between chlamydial infection and ectopic pregnancies through reduced tubal motility.

15.2.5 Prokinecticins

PROK1 and PROK2 are cognate ligands for the PROK1 and PROK2 receptors, and signalling through either PROK receptor is possible. PROKs are thought to have a role in tubal smooth muscle contraction [19]. PROK1 has been shown to increase COX-2 (cyclooxygenase) levels and thereby regulate prostaglandin production in the Fallopian tube, which in turn affects tubal smooth muscle contractility [20]. Reduced PROKR expression in women with ectopic pregnancies may explain the role of PROKS. A reduced PROKR mRNA has been observed in women with tubal ectopic pregnancies [21]. A second proposed theory is that a low serum human chorionic gonadotrophin (hCG) level (seen in ectopic pregnancies) is associated with low PROK1 levels. hCG is known to increase PROK1 expression in the endometrium and a similar effect may be possible in the Fallopian tube [22].

15.2.6 Endocannabinoids

The endocannabinoid receptor (CB1/CNR1) has been silenced in a murine model of ectopic pregnancy with the resultant effect of embryo retention within the Fallopian tube, an effect that can be reversed by adrenergic stimulation. This suggests a role of the CB1 receptor in tubal motility [23]. Low CB1 expression in the epithelial and smooth muscle layers of Fallopian tubes in women with ectopic pregnancies also highlights their role [24]. High nicotine levels (as in cigarette smoke) are known to alter the levels of endocannabinoids in rat brains. A similar effect has been observed in human Fallopian tubes and may explain the association between cigarette smoking and tubal ectopic pregnancies [25].

15.3 Role of the Tubal Microenvironment

15.3.1 Integrins

In the human uterus, a 'window of implantation' in the mid-luteal phase of the menstrual cycle has been described during which endometrial receptivity enables the apposition, adhesion and invasion of the embryo into the uterine wall (Table 15.2).

This window is associated with marked changes in integrin expression within the endometrial epithelium [26]. The markers for endometrial receptivity for the embryo include integrins – α1β1, α4β1 and αvβ3 – and in mice models functional blockade of αvβ3 is associated with reduced implantation rates [27]. The integrins are a family of heterodimeric cell surface receptors that mediate cell–cell and cell–extracellular matrix adhesion and are capable of transducing bidirectional signals across the cell membrane. The role of integrins in the development of tubal ectopic pregnancies is poorly understood due to limited evidence. Two semi-quantitative immunohistochemical studies have suggested a potential implantation window in the Fallopian tube, secondary to integrin marker expression, facilitating tubal implantation [28, 29]. However a newer, more comprehensive study revealed no evidence for changes in the expression or distribution of all five integrin receptivity markers (α1, α4, αV, β1 and β3) during the putative window of implantation in the mid-luteal phase of the cycle [30].

15.3.2 Uteroglobin

Uteroglobin is a low molecular weight peptide with anti-inflammatory properties and is produced by the secretory epithelial cells of the human Fallopian tube. Higher levels have been found in the Fallopian tubes of women with ectopic pregnancies and those with pelvic inflammatory disease (PID), which has been proposed to increase the receptivity of the Fallopian tube secondary to an altered anti-inflammatory effect and expression of factors associated with embryo implantation [31].

15.3.3 Leukaemia Inhibitory Factor (LIF)

LIF has been shown to be essential for implantation of mice embryos. PROKs are known to be associated with up-regulation of LIF [20, 22]. Higher levels of LIF have been demonstrated in ectopic implantation sites as compared to adjacent sites in the Fallopian tube. LIF expression in the Fallopian tube is noted to be higher in women with ectopic pregnancies and in chronic tubal inflammation [32]. Cigarette smoking and *Chlamydia* exposure may therefore increase PROKR expression and up-regulation of LIF, making the Fallopian tube receptive to embryo implantation and lead to ectopic pregnancies.

15.3.4 Mucin 1 (MUC1)

Mucin 1 is an anti-adhesive glycoprotein found in the female reproductive tract, which is thought to act as a barrier, preventing inappropriate embryo implantation in the Fallopian tube [33]. The human blastocyst induces removal of MUC1 and facilitates embryo implantation in in vitro studies [34]. Reduced MUC1 expression and altered glycosylation is noted in the Fallopian tube of women with ectopic pregnancy [35, 36].

15.3.5 Trophinin

Trophinin is a membrane protein which, when in complex with cytoplasmic proteins tastin and bystin, is thought to mediate adhesion between the embryo and the endometrium [37]. The Fallopian tube in women with tubal ectopic pregnancy shows a much higher expression of trophinin as compared to intrauterine pregnancies [38]. In addition, signalling from an embryo with arrested development in the Fallopian tube is thought to increase the expression of trophinin, tastin and bystin, contributing to greater tubal receptivity [38].

15.3.6 Activins

Activins are members of the TGF-β family of proteins and are formed by the dimerization of two inhibin β subunits. Three potential activin proteins exist: activin-A (βA-βA), activin-B (βB-βB) and activin-AB (βA-βB). Activin and activin receptor proteins are increased in women with tubal ectopic pregnancy as demonstrated using immunohistochemistry. In addition, activin-A expression is increased in women with tubal ectopic pregnancy who were serologically positive for *C. trachomatis* infection compared to those who are negative [18]. Activins are shown to play a role in endometrial decidualisaton, up-regulation of MMP expression and thereby implantation. Increased activin expression in the Fallopian tube (secondary to *C. trachomatis* infection) may enhance receptivity through tissue remodelling in the fallopian tube [39]. Activins also enhance NOS production [40], and increased activin expression may therefore alter tubal motility (smooth muscle contraction) and/or ciliary function, thereby predisposing to ectopic implantation.

15.3.7 Homeobox Protein A10

Homeobox protein A10 (HOXA10), a transcription factor, has been shown to be necessary for implantation in animal studies [41]. In women with tubal ectopic pregnancy, the expression of HOXA10 is shown to be higher at the implantation site within the Fallopian tube [42], suggesting a role for the embryo in its regulation/expression. This abnormal expression of HOXA10 is in turn thought to promote tubal implantation.

15.3.8 Interleukins

Interleukin (IL) 1 (IL-1) is produced by the embryo and is thought to regulate endometrial implantation [43]. IL-1 acts as a pro-inflammatory cytokine when produced by the tubal epithelium, in response to *C. trachomatis* infection. IL-1 induces production of IL-8 in this scenario. This inflammatory chemokine induces neutrophil-mediated tissue damage and this is in turn thought to promote tubal implantation [44].

15.3.9 Embryo Factor/E-Cadherin

There are several proposed mechanisms for development of a tubal ectopic pregnancy following IVF, although the aetiology still remains unclear. E-cadherin is a transmembrane glycoprotein and adhesion molecule, which is considered important for the development of the blastocyst and implantation in murine models. Embryos that lack E-cadherin expression fail to implant [45]. Revel et al. [46] demonstrated using immunohistochemistry that tubal implantation sites following IVF had a stronger expression of E-cadherin when compared to naturally conceived pregnancies. This expression was predominantly localised to the trophoblastic cells rather than the tubal epithelium. The authors hypothesise that the culture systems used for IVF are different from the natural environment conditions in vivo, and this may affect the development of the pre-implantation embryo. These embryos maybe 'non sticky' at the time of endometrial transfer (ET), and hence fail to implant in the receptive intrauterine environment with a resultant tubal ectopic pregnancy.

15.4 Role of the Tubal Immune cell – Embryo Interaction

15.4.1 Intra-Epithelial Lymphocytes

Intra-epithelial lymphocytes within the Fallopian tube are thought to prevent an immune response to the embryo during normal implantation [47]. ER-β expressing lymphocytes are found in higher numbers in women with tubal ectopic pregnancy suggesting a role in a disordered immune response.

15.4.2 Role of CD Cells

CD56bright CD16-NK cells are thought to regulate trophoblast invasion in part, during endometrial implantation [48]. These cells are absent in the Fallopian tube in an ectopic pregnancy, which is thought to be the reason for unregulated trophoblast invasion into the tube [49, 50]. CD56dim CD16neg cells are found in the Fallopian tube in ectopic pregnancies [51]. These cells lack cytotoxic properties, which are presented in the CD56dim found in peripheral blood [51, 52]. The absence of CD16 expression in the CD56dim cells in the tubal ectopic pregnancies and the subsequent lack of cytotoxicity is thought to be responsible for uncontrolled tubal trophoblastic invasion and absence of apoptosis. A number of other immune cell types (CD8pos lymphocytes, CD68pos macrophages, CD11cpos dendritic cells) are found in significantly higher numbers in the pregnant Fallopian tube, compared to the non-pregnant, suggesting a disordered signalling to the embryo due to an abnormal immune microenvironment in the Fallopian tube [49, 53].

15.4.3 Naturally Occurring Peptides

Secretory leucocyte protease inhibitor (SLPI) and elafin are expressed in the human Fallopian tube and are thought to offer immune protection of the tube during normal menstruation. They represent anti-protease and anti-microbial peptides, and an increased expression is seen in women with tubal ectopic pregnancy secondary to a *C. trachomatis* infection [54]. IL-1 may also increase the expression of elafin and SPLI in response to chlamydial infection [55, 56].

15.5 Role of the Tubal-Embryo Interactions and Angiogenesis

Vascular endothelial growth factor (VEGF) and placental growth factor (PlGF) have an important role to play in intrauterine implantation. The production of these angiogenic molecules occurs at the implantation site, and they act via specialised receptors [57–59].

15.5.1 Role of Vascular Endothelial Growth Factor

VEGF and its receptor (KDR) expression are higher at tubal ectopic implantation sites as compared to the remainder of the Fallopian tube [60]. There is close correlation between hCG and VEGF levels, suggesting a pattern of embryo-regulated vascularisation [60, 61]. Serum VEGF levels are found to be higher in women with tubal ectopic pregnancy as compared to intrauterine pregnancy [62]. Hypoxia at the tubal implantation site signals increased VEGF expression by the embryo [63]. VEGF in turn promotes local angiogenesis, increasing oxygen levels to the embryo and thereby promoting tubal implantation [64].

15.5.2 Role of Placenta Growth Factor

Serum PlGF levels are lower in women with tubal ectopic pregnancy as compared to intrauterine pregnancy [65]. PlGF is produced by the early trophoblast. Low PlGF mRNA and protein levels are identified in trophoblast isolates from tubal ectopic pregnancies as compared to intrauterine pregnancy [65]. Disordered embryo signalled angiogenesis at tubal implantation sites is thought to be responsible for this effect.

15.5.3 hCG Levels

Low hCG levels are the effect of an ectopic pregnancy. Serum bhCG assessments are based on the doubling time or 66 per cent rise in 48 hours in healthy pregnancies. However, 15 per cent of healthy IUPs do not increase by 66 per cent, 13 per cent of ectopic pregnancies have a 66 per cent rise in bhCG levels and 64 per cent of very early ectopic pregnancies may have doubling bhCG levels

15.6 Conclusion

Our current understanding of tubal ectopic pregnancies is limited to well-defined epidemiological risk factors; however, the exact underlying pathophysiological mechanisms remain unclear. Establishing a causal relationship to proposed mechanisms including events at a cellular level is difficult, as all tissue sampling occurs from women who have 'current' tubal ectopic pregnancies and is compared to tubal samples from non-pregnant women rather than tubal samples from healthy intrauterine pregnancies due to obvious practical and ethical constraints. Studies in animal models are also not a suitable alternative as a tubal ectopic pregnancy is an uncommon event in animals. However, further research into the aetiology of tubal ectopic pregnancies is essential to identify biomarkers for early diagnosis and other diagnostic tools, to identify risks factors and measures that might help prevent tubal ectopic pregnancies and to devise minimally invasive treatments with a view to preserving fertility and reducing morbidity.

Table 15.2 Summary of embryo-controlled factors in the aetiology of tubal ectopic pregnancy

Factor	Expression in the Fallopian tube of women with tubal ectopic pregnancy	Probable effect
Uteroglobin	Increased	Increased tubal receptivity
Leukaemia inhibitory factor (LIF)	Increased	Increased tubal receptivity
Homeobox protein A10 (HOXA 10)	Increased	Increased tubal receptivity
Vascular endothelial growth factor (VEGF)	Increased	Hypoxia-driven angiogenesis favouring a more receptive tubal microenvironment
Trophonin	Increased	Increased tubal embryo adhesion
Integrins	Increased	Increased tubal receptivity

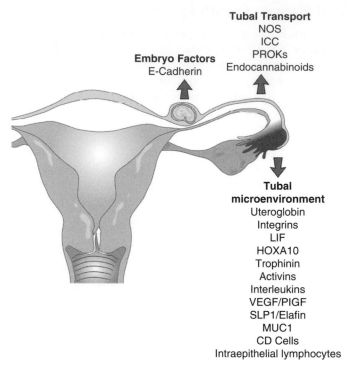

Tubal Transport
NOS
ICC
PROKs
Endocannabinoids

Embryo Factors
E-Cadherin

Tubal microenvironment
Uteroglobin
Integrins
LIF
HOXA10
Trophinin
Activins
Interleukins
VEGF/PIGF
SLP1/Elafin
MUC1
CD Cells
Intraepithelial lymphocytes

Figure 15.1 Aetiology of ectopic pregnancy

References

1. Brown JK, Horne AW. Laboratory models for studying ectopic pregnancy. *Curr Opin Obstet Gynecol.* 2011;23:221–6.

2. Varma R, Gupta J. Tubal ectopic pregnancy. *BMJ Clin Evid.* 2012 Feb;10:1406.

3. Corpa JM. Ectopic pregnancy in animals and humans. *Reproduction.* 2006;131:631–40.

4. Bouyer J, Coste J, Shojaei T et al. Risk factors for ectopic pregnancy: a comprehensive analysis based on a large case-control, population-based study in France. *Am J Epidemiol.* 2003;157:185–94.

5. Tay JI, Moore J, Walker JJ. Ectopic pregnancy. *BMJ.* 2000;320:916–9.

6. Pisarska MD, Carson SA, Buster JE. Ectopic pregnancy. *Lancet.* 1998;351: 1115–20.

7. Halbert S, Tam P, Blandau R. Egg transport in the rabbit oviduct: the roles of cilia and muscle. *Science.* 1976;191:1052–3.

8. Lyons R, Saridogan E, Djahanbakhch O. The reproductive significance of human Fallopian tube cilia. *Human Reproduction Update.* 2006;12:363–72.

9. Lyons RA, Saridogan E, Djahanbakhch O. The effect of ovarian follicular fluid and peritoneal fluid on Fallopian tube ciliary beat frequency. *Hum Reprod.* 2006;21: 52–6.

10. Paltieli Y, Eibschitz I, Ziskind G et al. High progesterone levels and ciliary dysfunction–a possible cause of ectopic pregnancy. *J Assist Reprod Genet.* 2000;17: 103–6.

11. Vasquez G, Winston RM, Brosens IA. Tubal mucosa and ectopic pregnancy. *Br J Obstet Gynaecol.* 1983;90:468–74.

12. McGee ZA, Jensen RL, Clemens CM et al. Gonococcal infection of human fallopian tube mucosa in organ culture: relationship of mucosal tissue TNF-alpha concentration to sloughing of ciliated cells. *Sex Transm Dis.* 1999;26:160–5.

13. Knoll M, Shaoulian R, Magers T, Talbot P. Ciliary beat frequency of hamster oviducts is decreased in vitro by exposure to solutions of mainstream and sidestream cigarette smoke. *Biol Reprod.* 1995;53:29–37.

14. Dixon RE, Hwang SJ, Hennig GW et al. Chlamydia infection causes loss of pacemaker cells and inhibits oocyte transport in the mouse oviduct. *Biol Reprod.* 2009;80:665–73.

15. Popescu LM, Ciontea SM, Cretoiu D. Interstitial Cajal-like cells in human uterus and fallopian tube. *Ann N Y Acad Sci.* 2007;1101:139–65.

16. Popescu LM, Ciontea SM, Cretoiu D et al. Novel type of interstitial cell (Cajal-like) in human fallopian tube. *J Cell Mol Med.* 2005;9:479–523.

17. Ekerhovd E, Norstrom A. Involvement of a nitric oxide-cyclic guanosine monophosphate pathway in control of fallopian tube contractility. *Gynecol Endocrinol.* 2004;19:239–46.

18. Refaat B, Al-Azemi M, Geary I, Eley A, Ledger W. Role of activins and inducible nitric oxide in the pathogenesis of ectopic pregnancy in patients with or without Chlamydia trachomatis infection. *Clin Vaccine Immunol.* 2009;16:1493–503.

19. Maldonado-Perez D, Evans J, Denison F, Millar RP, Jabbour HN. Potential roles of the prokinecticins in reproduction. *Trends Endocrinol Metab.* 2007;18:66–72.

20. Evans J, Catalano RD, Brown P et al. Prokineticin 1 mediates fetal-maternal dialogue regulating endometrial leukemia inhibitory factor. *FASEB J.* 2009;23:2165–75.

21. Shaw JL, Denison FC, Evans J et al. Evidence of prokineticin dysregulation in fallopian tube from women with ectopic pregnancy. *Fertil Steril.* 2010;94:1601–8 e1.

22. Evans J, Catalano RD, Morgan K et al. Prokineticin 1 signaling and gene regulation in early human pregnancy. *Endocrinology.* 2008;149:2877–87.

23. Wang H, Guo Y, Wang D et al. Aberrant cannabinoid signaling impairs oviductal transport of embryos. *Nat Med.* 2004;10:1074–80.

24. Horne AW, Phillips JA, 3rd, Kane N et al. CB1 expression is attenuated in Fallopian tube and decidua of women with ectopic pregnancy. *PLoS One.* 2008;3(12):e3969.

25. Gonzalez S, Cascio MG, Fernandez-Ruiz J et al. Changes in endocannabinoid contents in the brain of rats chronically exposed to nicotine, ethanol or cocaine. *Brain Res.* 2002;954:73–81.

26. Lessey B. Endometrial integrins and the establishment of uterine receptivity. *Human Reproduction.* 1998;13(suppl 3):247–58.

27. Illera MJ, Cullinan E, Gui Y et al. Blockade of the alpha(v)beta(3) integrin adversely affects implantation in the mouse. *Biol Reprod.* 2000;62:1285–90.

28. Makrigiannakis A, Karamouti M, Petsas G et al. The expression of receptivity markers in the fallopian tube epithelium. *Histochem Cell Biol.* 2009;132:159–67.

29. Sulz L, Valenzuela JP, Salvatierra AM, Ortiz ME, Croxatto HB. The expression of alpha(v) and beta3 integrin subunits in the normal human Fallopian tube epithelium suggests the occurrence of a tubal implantation window. *Hum Reprod.* 1998;13:2916–20.

30. Brown J, Shaw J, Critchley H, Horne A. Human fallopian tube epithelium constitutively expresses integrin endometrial receptivity markers: no evidence for a tubal implantation window. *Molecular Human Reproduction.* 2012;18:111–20.

31. Quintar AA, Mukdsi JH, del Valle Bonaterra M, et al. Increased expression of uteroglobin associated with tubal inflammation and ectopic pregnancy. *Fertil Steril.* 2008;89:1613–7.

32. Ji YF, Chen LY, Xu KH, Yao JF, Shi YF. Locally elevated leukemia inhibitory factor

in the inflamed fallopian tube resembles that found in tubal pregnancy. *Fertil Steril.* 2009;91:2308–14.

33. Gipson IK, Ho SB, Spurr-Michaud SJ et al. Mucin genes expressed by human female reproductive tract epithelia. *Biol Reprod.* 1997;56:999–1011.

34. Meseguer M, Pellicer A, Simon C. MUC1 and endometrial receptivity. *Mol Hum Reprod.* 1998;4:1089–98.

35. Al-Azemi M, Refaat B, Aplin J, Ledger W. The expression of MUC1 in human Fallopian tube during the menstrual cycle and in ectopic pregnancy. *Hum Reprod.* 2009;24:2582–7.

36. Savaris RF, da Silva LC, Moraes Gda S, Edelweiss MI. Expression of MUC1 in tubal pregnancy. *Fertil Steril.* 2008;89: 1015–7.

37. Aoki R, Fukuda MN. Recent molecular approaches to elucidate the mechanism of embryo implantation: trophinin, bystin, and tastin as molecules involved in the initial attachment of blastocysts to the uterus in humans. *Semin Reprod Med.* 2000;18:265–71.

38. Nakayama J, Aoki D, Suga T et al. Implantation-dependent expression of trophinin by maternal fallopian tube epithelia during tubal pregnancies: possible role of human chorionic gonadotrophin on ectopic pregnancy. *Am J Pathol.* 2003;163: 2211–19.

39. Dimitriadis E, White CA, Jones RL, Salamonsen LA. Cytokines, chemokines and growth factors in endometrium related to implantation. *Hum Reprod Update.* 2005;11:613–30.

40. Nusing RM, Barsig J. Induction of prostanoid, nitric oxide, and cytokine formation in rat bone marrow derived macrophages by activin A. *Br J Pharmacol.* 1999;127:919–26.

41. Bagot CN, Troy PJ, Taylor HS. Alteration of maternal Hoxa10 expression by in vivo gene transfection affects implantation. *Gene Ther.* 2000;7:1378–84.

42. Salih SM, Taylor HS. HOXA10 gene expression in human fallopian tube and

ectopic pregnancy. *Am J Obstet Gynecol.* 2004;190:1404–6.

43. Simon C, Pellicer A, Polan ML. Interleukin-1 system crosstalk between embryo and endometrium in implantation. *Hum Reprod.* 1995;10 Suppl 2:43–54.

44. Hvid M, Baczynska A, Deleuran B et al. Interleukin-1 is the initiator of Fallopian tube destruction during Chlamydia trachomatis infection. *Cell Microbiol.* 2007;9:2795–803.

45. Riethmacher D, Brinkmann V, Birchmeier C. A targeted mutation in the mouse E-cadherin gene results in defective preimplantation development. *Proceedings of the National Academy of Sciences.* 1995;92:855–9.

46. Revel A, Ophir I, Koler M, Achache H, Prus D. Changing etiology of tubal pregnancy following IVF. *Hum Reprod.* 2008;23:1372–6.

47. Kutteh WH, Blackwell RE, Gore H et al. Secretory immune system of the female reproductive tract. II. Local immune system in normal and infected fallopian tube. *Fertil Steril.* 1990;54:51–5.

48. Moffett-King A. Natural killer cells and pregnancy. *Nature Reviews Immunology.* 2002;2:656–63.

49. Shaw J, Fitch P, Cartwright J et al. Lymphoid and myeloid cell populations in the non-pregnant human Fallopian tube and in ectopic pregnancy. *Journal of Reproductive Immunology.* 2011;89:84–91.

50. von Rango U, Classen-Linke I, Kertschanska S, Kemp B, Beier HM. Effects of trophoblast invasion on the distribution of leukocytes in uterine and tubal implantation sites. *Fertility and Sterility.* 2001;76:116–24.

51. Laskarin G, Redzovic A, Vukelic P et al. Phenotype of NK cells and cytotoxic/ apoptotic mediators expression in ectopic pregnancy. *American Journal of Reproductive Immunology.* 2010;64:347–58.

52. Le Bouteiller P, Piccinni MP. REVIEW ARTICLE: Human NK cells in pregnant uterus: why there? *American Journal of Reproductive Immunology.* 2008;59:401–6.

53. Ulziibat S, Ejima K, Shibata Y et al. Identification of estrogen receptor β-positive intraepithelial lymphocytes and their possible roles in normal and tubal pregnancy oviducts. *Human Reproduction.* 2006;21:2281–9.

54. King AE, Wheelhouse N, Cameron S et al. Expression of secretory leukocyte protease inhibitor and elafin in human fallopian tube and in an in-vitro model of Chlamydia trachomatis infection. *Hum Reprod.* 2009;24:679–86.

55. King AE, Critchley HO, Kelly RW. Innate immune defences in the human endometrium. *Reprod Biol Endocrinol.* 2003;1:116.

56. Williams SE, Brown TI, Roghanian A, Sallenave JM. SLPI and elafin: one glove, many fingers. *Clin Sci (Lond).* 2006;110:21–35.

57. Plaisier M, Rodrigues S, Willems F et al. Different degrees of vascularization and their relationship to the expression of vascular endothelial growth factor, placental growth factor, angiopoietins, and their receptors in first-trimester decidual tissues. *Fertility and Sterility.* 2007;88:176–87.

58. Sugino N, Kashida S, Karube-Harada A, Takiguchi S, Kato H. Expression of vascular endothelial growth factor (VEGF) and its receptors in human endometrium throughout the menstrual cycle and in early pregnancy. *Reproduction.* 2002;123:379–87.

59. Torry DS, Leavenworth J, Chang M et al. Angiogenesis in implantation. *Journal of Assisted Reproduction and Genetics.* 2007;24:303–15.

60. Lam PM, Briton-Jones C, Cheung CK et al. Increased messenger RNA expression of vascular endothelial growth factor and its receptors in the implantation site of the human oviduct with ectopic gestation. *Fertil Steril.* 2004;82:686–90.

61. Torry DS, Torry RJ. Angiogenesis and the expression of vascular endothelial growth factor in endometrium and placenta. *American Journal of Reproductive Immunology.* 1997;37:21–9.

62. Felemban A, Sammour A, Tulandi T. Serum vascular endothelial growth factor as a possible marker for early ectopic pregnancy. *Hum Reprod.* 2002;17:490–2.

63. Shore VH, Wang TH, Wang CL et al. Vascular endothelial growth factor, placenta growth factor and their receptors in isolated human trophoblast. *Placenta.* 1997;18:657–65.

64. Daniel Y, Geva E, Lerner-Geva L et al. Levels of vascular endothelial growth factor are elevated in patients with ectopic pregnancy: is this a novel marker? *Fertility and Sterility.* 1999;72:1013–7.

65. Horne AW, Shaw JL, Murdoch A et al. Placental growth factor: a promising diagnostic biomarker for tubal ectopic pregnancy. *J Clin Endocrinol Metab.* 2011;96:E104–8.

Chapter 16

The Role of NK Cells in Implantation after IVF and Treatment Strategies

Dr Norman Shreeve and Ashley Moffett

16.1 Background

There are three types of lymphocyte, T cells, B cells and natural killer (NK) cells. T and B cells belong to the highly specific adaptive immune system, whereas NK cells are the lymphocytes of the innate immune system. In humans, a combination of the surface markers CD56 and CD16 identifies all the various subtypes of NK cells. NK cells in the blood (pbNK) recognize virally infected and cancerous cells, providing innate immunity through continuous peripheral surveillance. The name, natural killer, is derived from their ability to respond rapidly and lyse target cells in the absence of antibodies and human leukocyte antigen (HLA) molecules utilized by other lymphocytes. NK cells recognize either altered (e.g. virally stressed) or absent/foreign (e.g. allogeneic) expression of HLA on target cells through the identification of major histocompatibility complex (MHC) class I molecules (HLA in humans).

Cells belonging to the NK lineage exist in many organs, providing a wide and varying range of functional roles. Human NK cell populations are currently well described in the blood (majority are $CD56^{dim}CD16+$) and in a range of tissues, including lymph nodes, thymus, spleen, liver and uterus (uNK, $CD56^{superbright}CD16-$). It is important to note that whilst these cells probably originate from common progenitors, broad differences exist in the phenotypical markers and physiological roles between most tissue NK subtypes.

There are many mechanisms in humans and murine models that describe how mothers tolerate a genetically unfamiliar, invading conceptus. Since this notion of maternal tolerance to the semi-allogenic conceptus was first mooted, scientists and clinicians have described several ways that the fetal extra-villous trophoblast (EVT) can invade maternal tissue without triggering a response typical of allograft rejection. These include lack of expression of classical HLA molecules on trophoblast (HLA-A and HLA-B that are the dominant ligands for T cells); deviation of decidual antigen presenting cells (APCs) towards a tolerogenic phenotype by the trophoblast class I molecule HLA-G binding to the inhibitory receptor leukocyte immunoglobulin-like receptor subfamily B member 1 (LILRB1) on maternal APC; an abundance of regulatory T cells (Tregs) in the decidua; and expression of immune checkpoint inhibitors such as programmed cell death protein 1 (PD-1). It seems unlikely that all these mechanisms would fail at the same time in humans. Whilst mouse models have demonstrated that modifying maternal T cells can lead to fetal resorption, there are no convincing reports that any type of pregnancy failure in humans is due to effector T cells attacking the *placental trophoblast* cells. Evidence that maternal systemic T cells can and do respond to *fetal somatic* cells comes from the presence of antibodies to paternal HLA molecules (multiparous women were used as a source of these in the early days of tissue typing) and other allo-antigens expressed by red blood cells, platelets and so on. The mother is thus not generically tolerant to the fetus, but whether she does or does not display these allo-antibodies does not influence pregnancy outcome. The confusion in this area has come from (1) the failure to distinguish between systemic and local uterine T cell responses, (2) the failure to distinguish between extra-embryonic trophoblast and fetal somatic cells as the allogeneic cells and (3) the reliance on murine models despite the great differences in reproductive strategies between mice and humans.

Alongside this initial focus on T cells in human pregnancy, a significant field of investigation on the role of uNK has emerged. These were first identified by European anatomists early in the twentieth century and were described in 1921 as 'a type of lymphoid cell specific for the human decidua'. Following the discovery of NK cells in Sweden and the advent of immunohistology, 'uterine large granular lymphocytes' were described that were CD56^{bright}, CD16$^-$ by three groups in the United Kingdom in the 1990s [1]. The uNK are present in the non-pregnant endometrium where they proliferate following ovulation to become very abundant in the mid-late secretory phase. Around two days before menstruation, the uNK cells acquire an unusual appearance and die. This process has been little studied and deserves more attention because, as this is not seen in decidual NK, it is possible that endometrial NK contribute to the maintenance of the mucosa and prevent menstrual breakdown, possibly by secreting angiogenic factors that support the vasculature. The significance of this in IVF pregnancies is obvious as breakdown of the uterine mucosa following embryo transfer is common.

16.2 The Role of NK Cells in Implantation

The role of uNK at the stage where the blastocyst attaches to and invades the surface epithelium remains unclear. It is more likely that they play a role in the regulation of placentation, in particular the access of the placental cells to the uterine blood supply. During early pregnancy, uNK are the most abundant immune cell at the maternal-fetal interface, making up ~70 per cent of CD45+ cells. As a proportion of leukocytes, uNK levels drop towards term, pointing to a role in placental development. This early stage of pregnancy is critical in establishing an appropriate nutrient delivery to the fetus for organogenesis. It is at this stage that the remodelling of maternal spiral arteries by placental trophoblast cells takes place.

A clear demarcation line is drawn at the interface between the placenta (fetal origin) and the decidua (maternal origin) during placentation. The placental cells invade and transform the uterine arteries, establishing a high conductance blood supply. If this invasion is deficient, then when fetal demands become higher as gestation proceeds, the placenta (and fetus) can become 'starved' (Figure 16.1), with reduced fetal growth. Because the placental cells are fetal and express proteins encoded by paternal genes, they are allogeneic. Immune cells are the obvious type of cell that would have the ability to recognize and respond to these allogeneic placental cells. As described earlier, the ability of uterine T cells to respond to the placenta is limited.

However, NK cells are also capable of allo-recognition and do this by using germ-line-encoded receptors known as killer-like immunoglobulin receptors (KIRs). KIRs are a family of genes that show great diversity in human populations. Some members of the KIR family recognize highly polymorphic HLA class I molecules, especially HLA-C, which is the only classical HLA class I molecule expressed by the implanting placental cells. This means that

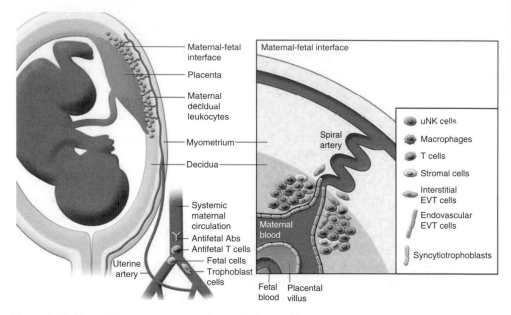

Maternal-fetal interface

Placenta

Maternal decidual leukocytes

Myometrium

Decidua

Systemic maternal circulation

Antifetal Abs

Antifetal T cells

Uterine artery

Fetal cells

Trophoblast cells

Maternal-fetal interface

Spiral artery

Maternal blood

Fetal blood

Placental villus

uNK cells

Macrophages

T cells

Stromal cells

Interstitial EVT cells

Endovascular EVT cells

Syncytiotrophoblasts

Figure 16.1 Maternal immune response to fetus and placenta [2]

each pregnancy is characterized by a woman with a certain set of KIR genes, combined with a baby that has inherited a particular HLA-C paternal ligand. Certain maternal KIR/fetal HLA-C genetic combinations can influence the outcome of pregnancy; for example, some are associated with pre-eclampsia and others with very large babies. The individual KIR genes differ by transmitting either an inhibitory or activating signal to the NK cell when bound to a cognate ligand. The overall balance of activating and inhibitory signals dictates the functional responses of the NK cell. Women who inherit strongly inhibitory KIR for HLA-C ligands are predisposed to disorders of placentation, whilst those with strongly activating KIR are more likely to have a large baby. In this way uNK cells subtly define the territorial boundary between the two different individuals, mother and her baby. KIR and HLA are immune system genes, and a recent computational modelling study suggests that the observed KIR allelic diversity and haplotypic organization in humans has been selected for by both responses to infections *and* reproductive fitness throughout evolution [3].

Experimental animal models have been key to our understanding of how uNK cells operate in the maternal decidua. Of particular use are studies utilizing those species who, like humans, employ a placental system where maternal blood directly contacts fetal tissue (haemochorial), e.g. mice, rats and guinea pigs. This bathing of the fetal chorion in maternal blood allows for efficient nutrient and gas exchange; however, it is likely to also provide a greater challenge to the mother's immune system. This is because placental cells penetrate the uterine wall to infiltrate the tissue, in contrast to the majority of species utilizing epitheliochorial placentae where the trophoblast merely sits on the surface epithelium.

Mice lacking uNK cells show normal implantation sites, suggesting that the key role these cells exert is not at this very early stage. In mice, uNK cells produce several substances that appear to be useful in promoting healthy placentation after successful implantation, e.g. vascular endothelial growth factor (VEGF) and interferon-gamma

(IFN-γ). As demonstrated in mouse models of pregnancy, IFN-γ is a key promotor of spiral artery remodelling [4] in the decidua, but an important mouse/human difference is that human uNK cells do not produce large amounts of IFN-γ. These species differences always need to be considered. Despite a lack of reliable modelling of trophoblast invasion in vitro, this process seems to be orchestrated by the production of interleukin-8 and interferon-inducible protein-10 chemokines [5]. However, of more relevance is the human genetic association data which have provided evidence that mothers who have a set of KIR genes encoding activating receptors are less likely to suffer gestational disorders of defective placentation, such as pre-eclampsia [6]. The soluble cytokines and chemokines produced by uNK suggest that uNK are critical in supporting normal human pregnancy, although exactly how they do this is unclear. To date there is no convincing evidence to suggest that uNK ever kill placental or fetal cells. When isolated from the uterus and challenged in vitro, these cells are poor killers of target cells and only become cytotoxic in the presence of interleukin-2, not normally present in the human uterus. There is thus absolutely no scientific basis at present to suggest uNK need 'suppressing'.

16.3 Measuring NK Cells in Assisted Reproductive Technology (ART)

It has been many years since initial descriptions of raised uNK activity in women with reproductive failure were published [6]. The continued use of assays to measure NK cells in the blood and the uterus in women with infertility or recurrent miscarriage is still highly controversial today. The reported increases in uNK cell numbers in recurrent miscarriage (RM) or recurrent implantation failure (RIF) during in vitro fertilization (IVF)/intra-cytoplasmic sperm injection (ICSI) have led to a surge in patients seeking pbNK and uNK cell measurements to explain their infertility. Treatment strategies based on these results are now extremely popular despite the complete lack of any underlying scientific rationale for their use and despite the potential risks of these treatments.

Despite their commercial success, these tests are highly problematic. Beyond proving clinical plausibility, many of these tests are yet to even undergo methodological validation. Neither is there a consensus on what should be considered a 'normal' number, with clinics often using vague figures of undefined cell populations. Variation between clinics exists as to what exactly 'normal' peripheral blood NK reference ranges are, even though it is known that values anywhere between 5 and 30 per cent of mononuclear cells should be considered in the normal range [7]. There is also no established consensus for 'normal' uNK number. Some studies have reported uNK numbers anything >5 per cent of stromal cells in the decidua as an 'abnormal' level [8]. Inconsistencies in this field have also arisen from varying sample timing in the menstrual cycle, studies lacking appropriately matched controls and the lack of a universal laboratory protocol for measuring uNK cell number or activity. This may in some part also reflect the significant heterogeneity in uNK cell number/cell-surface repertoire that exists between individuals. It is also not clear whether the numbers of NK cells present in the blood or uterus influences their functional capabilities – especially as there is still little certainty on what these are. Whilst techniques in flow cytometry (often used to measure NK numbers) are rapidly improving, until these issues are sufficiently addressed it seems that such measurements should not be used in clinical settings.

Assays to measure pbNK are rarely routinely used in any clinical condition apart from certain rare haematological disorders, because the clinical significance of the results is yet to be understood. As a result, blood samples taken in fertility clinics in the United Kingdom are commonly sent to Chicago for a range of 'immune' tests, including Th1/Th2 cytokine ratios, which are equally poorly understood. Treating otherwise healthy patients with immunosuppressive therapies, based on invalidated invasive tests, continues to cause concern among scientists, researchers and the mainstream media. Worryingly, a recent study of 233 HFEA-registered fertility treatment centres reported that many claims of benefit for interventions were not quantified and evidence not cited to support the claims [9]. Current advice from the Royal College of Obstetricians and Gynaecologists (2016) states: (1) 'there is no indication to offer routine uNK cell testing in women presenting with infertility or seeking IVF treatment'; and (2) 'women undergoing uNK cell testing should understand that there is, as yet, no proven effective treatment for those with what may be considered abnormal results' [10].

16.4 Preparing the Endometrial Immune Environment

Despite the lack of scientific rigour in this area, a number of adjunct immune therapies aimed at improving the success of IVF/ICSI cycles are currently in use. In the United Kingdom, these are generally confined to private healthcare settings and not subject to regulation by the HFEA. Whilst there are few NK cell-specific therapies available, much of the dogma surrounding maternal immune suppression in ART involves the concept of 'dampening' uNK cell activity in women suffering repeated early pregnancy loss or implantation failure. This logic stems entirely from an erroneous *belief* that NK cells may behave similarly to their cytotoxic counterparts in peripheral blood, and are harmful towards the invading trophoblast, resulting in pregnancy loss. Unlike religion, medical treatment cannot proceed on the basis of belief. There is no evidence that uNK cells are cytotoxic to the placenta or the fetus. A recent meta-analysis of 20 clinical trials involving various immune treatments for women with recurrent miscarriage showed that 'paternal cell immunization, third-party donor leukocytes, trophoblast membranes, and intravenous immunoglobulin provide no significant beneficial effect over placebo in improving the live birth rate' [11].

Thus, the use of presently available immune modulating agents in ART for improving pregnancy outcome is currently impossible to justify. Discussed below are some of the commonly used adjuncts purported to optimize the maternal immune system in favour of supporting pregnancy after IVF/ICSI.

16.4.1 Intravenous Immunoglobulin (IVIg)

This drug has a wide array of clinical uses, including in solid organ transplantation and in treating conditions characterized by antibody deficiencies. The rationale for its use in preventing early pregnancy loss remains unclear. It is clear that through Fc receptor blockade and complement neutralization, IVIg has the potential to down-regulate maternal immunity to potentially harmful pathogens. A recent multi-centred, randomized, double-blinded, placebo-controlled trial compared IVIg with saline in improving pregnancy success. The data from this study alone revealed that there was no benefit in administering IVIg to women with idiopathic secondary recurrent miscarriage. The authors *also* included two previous similar trials to conduct a separate meta-analysis, where again no benefit was reported [12]. The Department of Health currently includes 'recurrent spontaneous abortion' and 'IVF failure' as indications for which IVIg is *not* recommended. It is expensive and in short supply, so use in fit young women limits availability for seriously ill patients. It also has significant side effects and needs to be administered in a setting where there is adequate and immediate availability of the supportive medical care not usually found in a private clinic setting.

16.4.2 Intralipid

A fat-soluble soya-based lipid emulsion, Intralipid has numerous clinical utilities, including being widely used as a carrying media for anaesthetic agents and in cardiac protection after bupivacaine toxicity. It was first used in reproductive medicine when alternatives to the expensive and difficult-to-obtain IVIg became a problem. However, it is worth pointing out that Intralipid was actually used as the 'control' in a trial of another now discredited treatment for RM/IVF, paternal leukocyte immunization [13]. Its use in ART has become popular over recent years, especially in women suffering recurrent miscarriage or implantation failure, probably because it is cheap and its formulation as a white infusion has a powerful placebo effect. A recent double-blind randomized controlled trial (RCT) of 296 patients showed no clinical benefit in terms of chemical pregnancy rate 14 days after embryo transfer in women with a history of recurrent spontaneous abortion and the so-called 'raised' NK levels (>12 per cent – these are in fact within the normal range), who received Intralipid instead of a saline placebo [14]. The side effects can include infection secondary to intravenous cannulation, where atypical fungal organisms have been specifically associated with Intralipid infusions [15].

16.4.3 Glucocorticoids

Convincing clinical data to support the use of drugs such as prednisolone/dexamethasone in ART have also been hard to come by. Small cohort studies of patient subgroups (e.g. those with raised antinuclear antibodies, ANA, who have a disorder in the lupus spectrum) have shown some promise for adjuvant prednisolone in IVF/ICSI in improving blastocyst implantation rate; this group of patients with a specific auto-immune disease are clearly separate from most women attending IVF clinics. A large-scale meta-analysis [16] including data from 14 clinical trials where patients received peri-implantation glucocorticoids during their IVF or ICSI cycles revealed no benefit in terms of pregnancy rate. A subset analysis of those specifically undergoing IVF (and not ICSI) showed a borderline statistically significant improvement; however, the authors advise that these data be interpreted with care. These data were 'catch all' for routine glucocorticoid administration in ART, and should not necessarily be extrapolated to women with autoantibodies, unexplained infertility or recurrent implantation failure.

With a relatively low cost and high familiarity among patients, glucocorticoid regimes have become common within many infertility clinics. The concept relies upon the assumption that agents such as prednisolone dampen down an 'overactive' maternal immune system (measured through various NK assays) to achieve a more optimal endometrium for the fetal tissue to invade into. Notwithstanding the uncertain clinical efficacy, the significant immune suppression and well-described side effects associated with these drugs must be considered. Alongside the commonly recognized side effects (Table 16.1), there have been case reports of significant atypical maternal infectious disease associated with multiple immune suppression therapies during early pregnancy [17]. When considering that the vast majority of patients undergoing these treatments are medically well, potentially compromising their health with unproven interventions seems ill-advised.

Table 16.1 Summary of adjunctive immune therapies used in ART [20]

Drug	Common clinical uses	Side effects or adverse events
Lipid emulsion, e.g. *Intralipid* ©	Parenteral nutrition, administered with propofol, cardio-protection in bupivacaine toxicity	Hepatomegaly, jaundice, cholestasis, splenomegaly, thrombocytopenia, leukopenia and fat overload syndrome (<1 per cent occurrence in clinical trials)
Intravenous immunoglobulin (IVIg)	Primary and secondary antibody deficiency states, haematological disorders, neurological conditions, other uses, e.g. solid organ transplantation	Aseptic meningitis, renal failure, thromboembolism, haemolytic reactions, anaphylactic reactions, lung disease, enteritis, dermatologic disorders and infectious diseases
Corticosteroids	Suppression of inflammatory/allergic disorders, inflammatory bowel disease, asthma, croup, rheumatic disease, eye and ear conditions	Gastric ulceration, Cushing's syndrome, diabetes, hypocalcaemia, osteoporosis, skin thinning, dry skin, high blood sugar
Anti-tumour necrosis factor (Anti-TNF)	Autoimmune disorders, e.g. rheumatoid arthritis, ankylosing spondylitis, inflammatory bowel disease, psoriasis	Infection, lymphoma, demyelinating disease, autoantibody induction, congestive heart failure, injection site reactions, lupus-like syndrome
Granulocyte-colony stimulating factor (GM-CSF)	Neutropenia (various clinical types), severe or recurrent infections in advanced human immunodeficiency virus infection	Mucositis, splenic enlargement, hepatomegaly, transient hypotension, epistaxis, urinary abnormalities, osteoporosis, exacerbation of rheumatoid arthritis, anaemia, pseudogout

16.4.4 Anti-Tumour Necrosis Factor (TNF)

This class of anti-inflammatory drug is usually used to treat chronic inflammatory conditions such as rheumatoid arthritis and inflammatory bowel disease. It has been suggested that drugs within this class such as *Humira*© may improve pregnancy rates in patients with recurrent miscarriage and 'abnormal' immune profiles. This approach is based on earlier studies suggesting an association between recurrent miscarriage and raised TNF-alpha (TNF-α), an inflammatory cytokine. Small-scale uncontrolled trials have suggested a benefit in terms of pregnancy outcome in ART; however, there is a complete dearth of high-quality evidence to confirm these initial reports. Large-scale studies employed to detect the effects of anti-TNF in pregnancy among women receiving long-standing treatment have been more revealing. A study of nearly 2000 women in 2015 [18] suggested that TNF-α inhibitors may carry a risk of adverse pregnancy outcome of moderate clinical relevance with no improvement in the rate of spontaneous abortion. Because of these findings and the lack of evidence to support their use in infertility, the administration of these drugs should be confined to research settings only. The side effects of these treatments also need consideration.

16.4.5 GM-CSF

Granulocyte colony stimulating factor (GM-CSF) is a cytokine produced by many immune cells, including NK cells. As a broad leukocyte growth factor, it also has a key role in promoting the development of granulocytes and monocytes from haematopoietic stem cells. It is used in neutropenia prevention post-chemotherapy. In recent years, it has also been subject to extensive research as a potential adjunct in ART. A key study in 2013 suggested a potential therapeutic benefit for a related cytokine GM-CSF use when added to conventional embryo culture medium, as it increased embryo survival and live birth rate when compared to control media [19]. There is little evidence regarding its use as a maternal immune modulator *after* implantation however.

16.5 Future Directions

The best evidence for the role of uNK in reproductive success is the genetic evidence of combinations of NK KIR receptors with fetal HLA-C ligands. From this it appears that uNK cells regulate placentation following recognition of invading placental trophoblast cells. There is no direct contact of uNK with fetal cells. Perturbations in this early dialogue may increase the risk of life-threatening pregnancy complications, such as pre-eclampsia. As previously mentioned, the function of NK cells relies heavily upon the receptor-ligand interactions they constantly undergo. Other interactions between uNK and trophoblast and their influence on trophoblast and other cells in the decidua are also likely to be important. An important gap in our knowledge is how the trophoblast mediates destruction of the media of the spiral arteries and whether there are other uNK products that act directly to increase blood flow in the arteries. Lack of suitable animal models is a barrier to progress here, particularly the lack of human trophoblast cell lines. All NK cells are endowed with a highly polymorphic repertoire of inhibiting and activating receptors, including KIRs. How these NK receptors influence uNK functional abilities in pregnancy requires further experimental work. Of particular clinical importance may be the potential for large-scale human genetic association studies to uncover exactly which inhibitory KIR and HLA-C allelic combinations deliver high-risk pregnancy conditions, including miscarriage/implantation failure. Promising early data in oncology settings have revealed the potential for using monoclonal antibodies to block inhibitory KIR, resulting in a more potent innate immunity against cancerous cells. A similar approach in pregnancy may lead to the enhanced prediction of clinical conditions, and offer a novel approach for the development of KIR-specific therapeutic agents.

References

1. King A, Loke YW. On the nature and function of human uterine granular lymphocytes. *Immunol Today*. 1991;12:432–435.

2. Ashley Moffett, Francesco Colucci. Uterine NK cells: active regulators at the maternal-fetal interface. *J Clin Invest*. 2014 May 1; 124(5):1872–1879.

3. Penman Bridget S, Moffett Ashley, Chazara Olympe, Gupta Sunetra, Parham Peter. Reproduction, infection and killer-cell immunoglobulin-like receptor haplotype evolution. *Immunogenetics*. 2016; 68(10):755–764.

4. Ashkar AA, Croy BA. Functions of uterine natural killer cells are mediated by interferon gamma production during murine pregnancy. *Semin Immunol*. 2001 August;13(4): 235–41.

5. Hanna J, Goldman-Wohl D, Hamani Y et al. NK cells regulate key developmental processes at the human fetal-maternal

interface. *Nat Med.* 2006 September;12(9): 1065–74.

6. Hiby Susan E, Apps Richard, Andrew M et al. Maternal activating KIRs protect against human reproductive failure mediated by fetal HLA-C2. *J Clin Invest.* 2010 November 1; 120(11):4102–4110.

7. Bisset LR, Lung TL, Kaelin M, Ludwig E, Dubs RW. Reference values for peripheral blood lymphocyte phenotypes applicable to the healthy adult population in Switzerland. *Eur J Haematol.* 2004;72:203–12.

8. Quenby S, Kalumbi C, Bates M, Farquharson R, Vince G. Prednisolone reduces preconceptual endometrial natural killer cells in women with recurrent miscarriage. *Fertil Steril.* 2005;84:980–984.

9. Spencer EA, Mahtani KR, Goldacre B, Heneghan C. Claims for fertility interventions: a systematic assessment of statements on UK fertility centre websites. *BMJ Open.* 2016 November 27;6(11): e013940.

10. Laird SM. The Role of Natural Killer Cells in Human Fertility (Scientific Impact Paper No. 53). Published 28/11/16. Available at URL: www.rcog.org.uk/globalassets/docu ments/guidelines/scientific-impact-papers /sip_53.pdf. Accessed on 01/ 01/2017.

11. Wong LF, Porter TF, Scott JR. Immunotherapy for recurrent miscarriage. *Cochrane Database Syst Rev.* 2014 October 21;(10):CD000112.

12. Stephenson MD, Kutteh WH, Purkiss S et al. Intravenous immunoglobulin and idiopathic secondary recurrent miscarriage: a multicentered randomized placebo-controlled trial. *Hum Reprod.* 2010 September;25(9):2203–9.

13. Johnson PM, Ramsden GH, Chia KV et al. A combined randomised double-blind and open study of trophoblast membrane infusion (TMI) in unexplained recurrent miscarriage. In: ChaouatG, MowbrayJ editor(s). *Cellular molecular biology of the materno-fetal relationship.* Vol. 212,

Colloque IN- SERM/John Libbey Eurotext Ltd, 1991:277–84.

14. Dakhly DM, Bayoumi YA, Sharkawy M et al. Intralipid supplementation in women with recurrent spontaneous abortion and elevated levels of natural killer cells. *Int J Gynaecol Obstet.* 2016 December;135 (3):324–327.

15. Public Health England. UK Standards for Microbiology Investigations. Investigation of Intravascular Cannulae and Associated Specimens. Available at www.gov.uk/gov ernment/uploads/system/uploads/attach ment_data/file/518825/B_20dp_.pdf

16. Boomsma CM, Keay SD, Macklon NS. Peri-implantation glucocorticoid administration for assisted reproductive technology cycles. *Cochrane Database Syst Rev.* 2012 June 13;(6):CD005996.

17. Akhanoba F, MacDougall J, Mathur R, Hassan W. Severe systemic candidiasis following immunomodulation therapy in in vitro fertilisation-embryo transfer (IVF-ET). *BMJ Case Rep* 2014;2014:1–4.

18. Weber-Schoendorfer C, Oppermann M, Wacker E, Bernard N; network of French pharmacovigilance centres, Beghin D, Cuppers-Maarschalkerweerd B, Richardson JL, Rothuizen LE, Pistelli A, Malm H, Eleftheriou G, Kennedy D, Kadioglu Duman M, Meister R, Schaefer C. Pregnancy outcome after TNF-α inhibitor therapy during the first trimester: a prospective multicentre cohort study. *Br J Clin Pharmacol.* 2015 October;80(4): 727–39.

19. Ziebe S, Loft A, Povlsen BB et al. A randomized clinical trial to evaluate the effect of granulocyte-macrophage colony-stimulating factor (GM-CSF) in embryo culture medium for in vitro fertilization. *Fertil Steril.* 2013 May;99(6): 1600–9.

20. Moffett A, Shreeve N. First do no harm: uterine natural killer (NK) cells in assisted reproduction. *Hum Reprod.* 2015 July;30 (7):1519–25.

Sex and Immune Receptivity for Embryo Transfer

David J. Sharkey and Sarah A. Robertson

17.1 Introduction

An important aspect of endometrial receptivity for implantation is the female immune response. Remarkably, a couple's sexual activity and the male partner's seminal fluid appear to be important in preparing the female immune response to support embryo implantation. In the past, the male partner's contribution to reproduction has been thought to start and finish with providing sperm to fertilize the egg. His seminal fluid has been viewed simply as a transport and survival medium for spermatozoa to traverse the female reproductive tract and fertilize the oocyte. However, there is growing evidence that seminal fluid plays a more complex role, directly promoting fertility and fecundity through effects on the woman's immune response and her reproductive processes [1].

This has led to the question of whether sexual intercourse might be beneficial for the chances of conception and pregnancy in assisted reproduction treatment cycles. While sufficiently powered clinical studies to provide conclusive evidence are lacking, a recent meta-analysis of several small studies shows a benefit of sexual intercourse or assisted delivery of seminal fluid on conception rates in in vitro fertilization (IVF) embryo transfer (ET) cycles [2]. Studies of the physiological response of female tissues to seminal fluid reveal that at a biological level this operates through transmitting antigens and immune-regulatory factors, and inducing expression of genes and microRNAs, that together prepare the female immune response for pregnancy [1].

While intercourse during an IVF/ET cycle is clearly not essential for pregnancy after IVF conception, advocating abstinence around the time of ET and the resultant lack of immune priming may be counteractive to achieving pregnancy. Encouraging coitus where appropriate appears to be a safe, simple and low-cost way of improving the chances of success. This chapter will examine the current evidence as to whether seminal fluid delivers a beneficial effect on conception rates and will summarize our current understanding of the mechanisms by which it influences the female immune response. We argue that on balance the evidence supports a positive impact of seminal fluid around the time of ET.

17.2 Seminal Fluid Signalling and Immune Receptivity for Pregnancy

Seminal plasma, the fluid portion of semen produced primarily by the male accessory sex glands, contains abundant bioactive signalling agents that exert biological effects on female tissues. These agents include cytokines such as transforming growth factor beta (TGFB), prostaglandins of the E series and steroid hormones oestrogen and progesterone, all of which have established roles in immune regulation.

Most of our knowledge of the effects of seminal fluid comes from studies in animals, where comparable effects are shown in all mammals and even in invertebrate species. In rodents, where the post-mating inflammatory response has been extensively characterized, seminal fluid triggers a series of immune mechanisms that result in maternal immune tolerance to paternal transplantation antigens that are later expressed by the developing placenta and fetus [3]. The cytokines released during this response promote embryo development and successful implantation, while the immune cells suppress inflammation and facilitate robust placental development [1]. A critical consequence is stimulation of immune cells called regulatory T cells (or 'Treg cells'), which react with paternal transplantation antigens in seminal fluid and later expressed by the conceptus. These Treg cells have anti-inflammatory and immune-suppressive functions, and ensure optimal immune tolerance for pregnancy is established [4]. When pregnancy in mice is initiated in the absence of seminal fluid, through surgical removal of the male seminal vesicle glands, fertility and fecundity is reduced and the resultant offspring show signs of growth restriction and altered metabolic phenotype [5].

There is now substantial data that similar immune priming events are active in women after seminal fluid transmission at coitus [1]. The primary site within the human female reproductive tract to respond to seminal fluid is the cervix. In 1985, Pandya and Cohen were the first to demonstrate an efflux of leukocytes into cervical mucus following donor insemination with whole semen [6]. An equivalent inflammatory response was not observed when women were instead inseminated with sperm-free seminal plasma. In 1992, Thompson and colleagues used immunohistochemistry to identify neutrophils, and smaller numbers of macrophages and lymphocytes, as the main cell types recruited into the cervical mucus following artificial insemination [7]. The efflux of neutrophils into the cervical lumen is believed to be important for clearance of non-fertilizing sperm and cellular debris as well as for the prevention of infection by potentially harmful pathogens introduced at coitus.

In 2012, we published the first evidence that seminal fluid exposure following vaginal intercourse initiates an inflammation-like response within the ectocervix of periovulatory women. Immunohistochemical analysis of cervical tissue biopsies collected before and after unprotected intercourse identified macrophages and dendritic cells as predominant leukocyte populations recruited into the cervical epithelium and deeper stromal tissue following seminal fluid contact. Accumulation of a smaller contingent of lymphocytes, mostly of a memory T cell phenotype, was also observed. We found that leukocyte recruitment is regulated by seminal fluid induction of pro-inflammatory cytokines and chemokines including CSF2 (GM-CSF), IL6 and CXCL8. No inflammatory response was observed in the absence of intercourse or when seminal fluid contact was prevented using condoms [8]. This response indicates evidence of immune activation that we believe, based on our preclinical work, can boost the T cell reservoir that is then available for recruitment into the endometrium to facilitate the decidual response, embryo implantation and early placental development [1].

Whether direct, local effects of seminal fluid contact extend to the endometrium and fallopian tube remains to be determined. In vitro experiments show epithelial cells from these sites are capable of responding to components of seminal fluid by producing cytokines that can assist embryo development and pregnancy progression. In women, seminal fluid is mainly retained in the cervix, with cervical mucus selectively releasing populations of sperm that ascend to the uterus and fallopian tube to fertilize the oocyte. Transport mechanisms by which sperm and microparticles of seminal plasma can access the higher regions of the tract have been described. Firstly, rhythmic uterine peristaltic contractions may act to propel seminal fluid into the uterus and fallopian tube [9]. Secondly, TGFB, a key bioactive signalling agent in seminal fluid, has been shown to bind to the sperm surface and so could be carried by sperm to gain access to the endometrium [10]. It is also possible that seminal fluid constituents deposited in the vagina access the uterus via local countercurrent transfer from the vaginal venous blood, and possibly afferent lymphatics, into the uterine arterial blood. While these mechanisms reasonably could allow seminal fluid constituents to gain access to the higher female tract, whether seminal fluid-induced changes occur at the epithelial surface of the uterus and fallopian tube has not yet been reported.

17.3 Effect of Seminal Fluid Exposure around the Time of Embryo Transfer on IVF/ET Conception Rates

It is not uncommon for couples undergoing IVF/ET to refrain from sexual activity around the time of ET. The reasons are complex and varied. Patients may fear that the physical act of intercourse or uterine contractions associated with female orgasm could impede the transferred embryo from implanting successfully. Women and men may also have reduced libido associated with the physical and psychological challenges of treatment cycles. Doctors may actively discourage couples from intercourse due to the small but real risk of introducing infection into the higher female tract, at a time when the tract is vulnerable because of the recent breaching of the cervical mucus barrier by the ET catheter. Some clinicians express a concern of super-fecundity, where multiple pregnancies could result from natural and IVF conception – however, the risk of this seems small in infertile couples and should be mitigated by complete oocyte retrieval.

Interest in the possibility of benefits of seminal fluid contact is not new, and studies to investigate this stretch back at least to the 1980s. Around a dozen small studies of variable quality have addressed the impact of seminal fluid transmission either by intercourse or by assisted delivery to the vagina, cervix or uterus. The studies also differ in the nature of the control treatment (abstinence, no treatment or saline), whether fresh or frozen embryos are transferred and the outcomes measured. None of these studies was appropriately powered to prove benefit; however, almost all have shown small changes on conception rate, and in some cases live birth rate.

One of the earliest clinical studies involved couples undergoing IVF conception or gamete intra-fallopian transfer (GIFT) treatment. In this setting, intra-vaginal application of seminal plasma at around the time of embryo or gamete transfer was found to significantly improve live-birth rates [11]. Additionally, vaginal administration of pessaries prepared from pooled donor seminal plasma was reported to improve the likelihood of successful pregnancy in women experiencing recurrent miscarriage [12].

Two studies have specifically examined the effect of intercourse around the time of ET. In 2000, Tremellen and colleagues reported data from 600 women at two sites, including frozen ET in Australia and fresh cycles in Spain. Couples had intercourse either once within the 48-hour period prior to or after transfer (in frozen cycles) or just after ET (in fresh cycles), while the control group abstained. The study revealed a clear benefit of intercourse in the two days either before or after ET, with an approximate 50 per cent improvement in clinical implantation rate observed, compared to couples who abstained [13].

A second study performed in Iran in 2009 by Aflatoonian and colleagues examined the effect of intercourse on pregnancy rates in 390 women with a history of >5 years infertility who were undergoing either IVF or intracytoplasmic sperm injection (ICSI) cycles. Intercourse at least once in the 12-hour period following ET (all fresh cycles) resulted in an 18 per cent increase in implantation rate and a 21 per cent improvement in clinical pregnancy rates, when compared to women who abstained for the entire IVF/ICSI cycle, though these changes did not reach statistical significance [14].

Other studies have investigated transfer of whole semen or seminal plasma by artificial means. In 1986, Bellinge and colleagues performed a prospective study in 152 women undergoing IVF cycles for any form of infertility, to evaluate whether artificial instillation of the conceiving male partner's whole semen into the vagina in the 36- to 48-hour period prior to ET improved implantation rates. The authors reported a striking effect of vaginal insemination with whole semen, with an implantation rate of 53 per cent observed in inseminated women compared to just 23 per cent in women who were not [11]. In 2013, Chicea and colleagues examined whether instillation of the male partner's seminal plasma into the cervical canal and vagina after ovum pick-up (OPU) improved pregnancy rates following ET in 346 women undergoing IVF cycles. Women exposed to seminal plasma had significantly improved implantation rates compared to control women (34.7% vs. 27.5 per cent respectively, $p=0.026$). A trend towards an increase in clinical pregnancy rates was observed after seminal plasma treatment, compared to controls (55.5 per cent vs. 44 per cent respectively, $p=0.09$) [15]. Friedler and colleagues performed a similar study where the partner's seminal plasma was applied to the vaginal vault just after OPU in 220 couples undergoing either IVF or ICSI cycles with at least one previous failed IVF/ET attempt. A 26.8 per cent improvement in clinical pregnancy rate was observed following ET in women exposed to seminal plasma, compared to women given placebo. This is the only study wherein transfer of seminal plasma by artificial means increased the ongoing pregnancy rate (OPR). A 44 per cent relative increase in OPR was observed with seminal plasma treatment compared to placebo [(OPR) of 32.0 per cent (33/103) and 22.2 per cent (26/117), respectively] [16].

In 2015, Crawford and colleagues performed a meta-analysis of 2,204 patients encompassing a total of seven random controlled trials, where effects of seminal fluid exposure either by vaginal intercourse or by intravaginal, intracervical or intrauterine administration were evaluated. The meta-analysis revealed a clear benefit of seminal fluid exposure, with a 23 per cent improvement in clinical pregnancy rate observed [2]. Unfortunately, no firm conclusion on the effects of seminal fluid exposure on live birth rates could be made since this additional data were available for just two of the seven studies included [2].

Only one study in the meta-analysis failed to demonstrate an improvement in IVF conception rates following exposure to seminal fluid at around the time of ET [17]. In this study, women were administered a preparation of diluted seminal plasma into the uterine cavity at the time of oocyte retrieval and clinical pregnancy rates were compared to women receiving a saline placebo. The lack of effect of seminal fluid exposure contrasted with the authors' previous findings demonstrating a clear improvement in IVF conception rates following instillation of seminal plasma into the higher vagina, in close proximity to the cervix, following OPU [18]. This raises the prospect that the site of seminal fluid contact may be an important determinant of whether a beneficial effect on IVF conception rate is achieved. There is also the possibility that data are confounded by lack of compliance in control abstain groups, with seminal fluid exposure also occurring via intercourse.

On the balance of evidence, a beneficial effect of seminal fluid exposure on IVF conception is indicated by the clinical studies to date. Although the studies are not sufficiently powered to draw firm conclusions, it is notable that the largest effects are noted with whole seminal fluid transmission achieved by intercourse [13] or practitioner delivery [11]. Additionally, most studies to date have been timed to deliver seminal fluid around the time of oocyte retrieval or before ET, with only a couple including seminal fluid contact in the post ET or implantation phase.

At this time, there is insufficient data to determine from the clinical studies whether the cycle stage at seminal fluid contact is important. However, on the basis of laboratory studies investigating the responsiveness of female tissues according to hormone status, it seems likely that the effects of seminal fluid would be maximized in the peri-ovulatory phase compared to the luteal phase.

Additionally, the clinical studies to date vary in terms of the composition of seminal fluid delivered – some have used whole semen, while others use seminal plasma. Our studies in mice indicate that maximum impact on the female immune response is achieved with whole seminal fluid containing sperm and seminal plasma [19], and in vivo and in vitro studies point to the same conclusion for women [6–8].

17.4 Seminal Fluid and Impact on Gestational Disorders

As well as effects on IVF conception rates, there is evidence that regular seminal fluid contact affords a level of protection against gestational disorders in both spontaneously conceived and assisted conception pregnancies. Pregnancies initiated in the absence of contact with the conceiving partner's seminal fluid, as occurs with donor gametes, are at greater risk of being complicated by gestational hypertension and pre-eclampsia [20]. In this setting, a lack of prior exposure to the conceiving partner's seminal fluid is thought to result in impaired placental development secondary to a deficient maternal immune to paternal antigens [21]. The elevated risk of developing gestational disorders using donor sperm is alleviated by multiple prior insemination cycles, but only when seminal fluid is from the same donor [22].

In women with azoospermic partners where sperm retrieval by testicular aspiration and fertilization via ICSI is necessary, the incidence of pre-eclampsia is threefold higher compared to IVF- or ICSI-initiated pregnancies using ejaculated sperm [23].

An increased risk of pre-eclampsia is also observed in spontaneously conceived pregnancies initiated after limited sexual contact, either as a result of a short period of sexual cohabitation or through the use of barrier methods of contraception. These observations also support a cumulative benefit of exposure to the conceiving partner's semen. The incidence of fetal growth restriction and pre-eclampsia in spontaneously conceived pregnancies is inversely related to duration of sexual relationship, with protection conferred after greater than three months of regular sexual cohabitation [24]. The reduced risk of developing pre-eclampsia afforded by prolonged seminal fluid exposure is consistent with 'priming' and strengthening of the female immune response. Importantly, the beneficial effects of seminal fluid exposure on pregnancy outcome appear to be partner-specific, with previous protection from the development of gestational disorders lost when a change in conceiving male partner has occurred [20].

The mechanism linking prolonged seminal fluid exposure with reduced likelihood of developing gestational disorders of pregnancy is believed to have a basis in immunological memory mediated by T cells. Repeated contact with the same seminal fluid antigens acts to prime and boost the adaptive immune response, causing progressive expansion in the pool of immune cells available for recruitment into the cervical and endometrial tissues to drive maternal immune preparation for pregnancy.

17.5 Variation in Seminal Fluid Composition – a Determinant of Fertility?

There are differences in the immune stimulatory capacity of seminal fluid between men – even amongst those with proven fertility – that can be measured as the capacity to stimulate synthesis of cytokines in cervical epithelial cells in vitro [25]. Men who are partners of women with unexplained infertility and repeated miscarriage can exhibit specific changes in seminal fluid constituents [26]. These differences raise the possibility that the relative amounts of signalling agents in seminal fluid have important consequences for male fertility status. The diagnostic utility of measuring seminal fluid cytokines as biomarkers of fertility, as an addition to measuring conventional sperm parameters, is under development and may soon become an addition to male fertility work-up.

There are several active constituents in human seminal fluid that influence the female tract immune response. In 2012, we identified the three mammalian isoforms of TGFB (TGFB1, TGFB2 and TGFB3) as key mediators of seminal fluid signalling. TGFB acts by inducing expression of potent immune-regulatory and pro-tolerance genes CSF2 and IL6 [27]. Prostaglandins of the E series, particularly the hydroxylated forms of PGE1 and PGE2, are also abundant in seminal fluid and induce CXCL8 production in cervical tissue explants in vitro [28]. In addition to its likely tolerance-inducing role, high concentrations of prostaglandins in seminal fluid may help to protect the male gametes from oxidative and inflammatory damage. The male microbiome may contribute to seminal fluid signalling as bacterial products like LPS are present in seminal fluid, and attenuate cytokine production in female tract cells [29]. Seminal fluid also contains HLA-G, which is produced by the testis and epididymis and is implicated in promoting tolerance in female tissues [30].

Importantly, some agents in seminal plasma can suppress the female tract response to seminal fluid. Recently, we have identified IFNG as a potent inhibitor of TGFB signalling in cervical epithelial cells [31]. IFNG levels are highly variable between men and also fluctuate within men over time, and may relate to the microbiome and other environmental factors [29]. In particular, studies showing elevated IFNG in partners of women with unexplained infertility are consistent with a key role for this factor in suppressing seminal fluid immune priming. However, IFNG in seminal fluid can be counteracted at least partly by high TGFB content [31]. Thus, it seems that the relative balance of different constituent factors in seminal plasma is important, and diagnostic tests for seminal fluid immune-regulatory function will need to reflect this.

17.6 Conclusions

In summary, there is growing evidence that encouraging couples to have sexual intercourse before or around the time of ET may have benefits for IVF/ET success. The evidence to date, although of limited quality because of the size and variable design of studies, can be interpreted to show that seminal fluid contact in an IVF/ET cycle improves the chances of implantation and has no overt adverse impact. Additional data implicates cumulative exposure prior to a conception cycle as facilitating healthy pregnancy progression with protection from pre-eclampsia and IUGR. Laboratory-based research in animals and human tissues provides compelling evidence that effects of seminal fluid are mediated through activating a female immune response that supports implantation and pregnancy progression. On the basis of this, we argue that there is little risk and a degree of benefit to be gained from recommending that, if possible, couples have intercourse before or around the time of ET. There is now an imperative to undertake large, well-designed studies to evaluate the relative importance of sexual intercourse as opposed to assisted delivery of seminal fluid, whether seminal plasma is sufficient or whole semen is required, the timing of the treatment cycle at which seminal fluid contact delivers the greatest benefit, and the extent of benefit in fresh versus frozen cycles.

References

1. Robertson SA, Sharkey DJ. Seminal fluid and fertility in women. *Fertil Steril* 2016;106:511–519.

2. Crawford G, Ray A, Gudi A, Shah A, Homburg R. The role of seminal plasma for improved outcomes during in vitro fertilization treatment: review of the literature and meta-analysis. *Hum Reprod Update* 2015;21:275–284.

3. Robertson SA, Guerin LR, Bromfield JJ et al. Seminal fluid drives expansion of the CD4+CD25+ T regulatory cell pool and induces tolerance to paternal alloantigens in mice. *Biol Reprod* 2009;80:1036–1045.

4. Guerin LR, Moldenhauer LM, Prins JR et al. Seminal fluid regulates accumulation of FOXP3+ regulatory T cells in the preimplantation mouse uterus through expanding the FOXP3+ cell pool and CCL19-mediated recruitment. *Biol Reprod* 2011;85:397–408.

5. Bromfield JJ, Schjenken JE, Chin PY et al. Maternal tract factors contribute to paternal seminal fluid impact on metabolic phenotype in offspring. *Proc Natl Acad Sci USA* 2014;111:2200–2205.

6. Pandya IJ, Cohen J. The leukocytic reaction of the human uterine cervix to spermatozoa. *Fertil Steril* 1985;43:417–421.

7. Thompson LA, Barratt CL, Bolton AE, Cooke ID. The leukocytic reaction of the human uterine cervix. *Am J Reprod Immunol* 1992;28:85–89.

8. Sharkey DJ, Tremellen KP, Jasper MJ, Gemzell-Danielsson K, Robertson SA. Seminal fluid induces leukocyte recruitment and cytokine and chemokine mRNA expression in the human cervix after coitus. *J Immunol* 2012;188:2445–2454.

9. Kunz G, Beil D, Deininger H, Wildt L, Leyendecker G. The dynamics of rapid sperm transport through the female genital tract: evidence from vaginal sonography of uterine peristalsis and hysterosalpingoscintigraphy. *Hum Reprod* 1996;11:627–632.

10. Chu TM, Nocera MA, Flanders KC, Kawinski E. Localization of seminal plasma transforming growth factor-beta1 on human spermatozoa: an immunocytochemical study. *Fertil Steril* 1996;66:327–330.

11. Bellinge BS, Copeland CM, Thomas TD et al. The influence of patient insemination on the implantation rate in an in vitro fertilization and embryo transfer program. *Fertil Steril* 1986;46:252–256.

12. Coulam CB, Stern JJ. Effect of seminal plasma on implantation rates. *Early Pregnancy* 1995;1:33–36.

13. Tremellen KP, Valbuena D, Landeras J et al. The effect of intercourse on pregnancy rates during assisted human reproduction. *Hum Reprod* 2000;15:2653–2658.

14. Aflatoonian A, Ghandi S, Tabibnejad N. The effect of intercourse around embryo transfer on pregnancy rate in assisted reproductive technology cycles. *Int J Fertil Steril* 2009;2:169–172.

15. Chicea R, Ispasoiu F, Focsa M. Seminal plasma insemination during ovum-pickup –a method to increase pregnancy rate in IVF/ICSI procedure. A pilot randomized trial. *J Assist Reprod Genet* 2013;30:569–574.

16. Friedler S, Ben-Ami I, Gidoni Y et al. Effect of seminal plasma application to the vaginal vault in in vitro fertilization or intracytoplasmic sperm injection treatment cycles-a double-blind, placebo-controlled, randomized study. *J Assist Reprod Genet* 2013;30:907–911.

17. von Wolff M, Rosner S, Germeyer A et al. Intrauterine instillation of diluted seminal plasma at oocyte pick-up does not increase the IVF pregnancy rate: a double-blind, placebo controlled, randomized study. *Hum Reprod* 2013;28:3247–3252.

18. von Wolff M, Rosner S, Thone C et al. Intravaginal and intracervical application of seminal plasma in in vitro fertilization or intracytoplasmic sperm injection treatment cycles–a double-blind, placebo-controlled, randomized pilot study. *Fertil Steril* 2009;91:167–172.

19. Guerin LR, Prins JR, Robertson SA. Regulatory T-cells and immune tolerance in pregnancy: a new target for infertility treatment? *Hum Reprod Update* 2009;15:517–535.

20. Dekker G. The partner's role in the etiology of preeclampsia. *J Reprod Immunol* 2002;57:203–215.

21. Redman CW. Pre-eclampsia: Definitions, paternal contributions and a four stage model. *Pregnancy Hypertens* 2011;1:2–5.

22. Kyrou D, Kolibianakis EM, Devroey P, Fatemi HM. Is the use of donor sperm associated with a higher incidence of preeclampsia in women who achieve pregnancy after intrauterine insemination? *Fertil Steril* 2010;93:1124–1127.

23. Wang JX, Knottnerus A-M, Schuit G et al. Surgically obtained sperm, and risk of gestational hypertension and pre-eclampsia. *The Lancet* 2002;359:673–674.

24. Kho EM, McCowan LM, North RA et al. Duration of sexual relationship and its effect on preeclampsia and small for gestational age perinatal outcome. *J Reprod Immunol* 2009;82:66–73.

25. Sharkey DJ, Macpherson AM, Tremellen KP, Robertson SA. Seminal plasma differentially regulates inflammatory cytokine gene expression in human cervical and vaginal epithelial cells. *Mol Hum Reprod* 2007;13:491–501.

26. Havrylyuk A, Chopyak V, Boyko Y, Kril I, Kurpisz M. Cytokines in the blood and semen of infertile patients. *Cent Eur J Immunol* 2015;40:337–344.

27. Sharkey DJ, Macpherson AM, Tremellen KP et al. TGF-beta mediates proinflammatory seminal fluid signaling in human cervical epithelial cells. *J Immunol* 2012;189:1024–1035.

28. Denison FC, Calder AA, Kelly RW. The action of prostaglandin E2 on the human cervix: stimulation of interleukin 8 and inhibition of secretory leukocyte protease inhibitor. *Am J Obstet Gynecol* 1999;180:614–620.

29. Sharkey DJ, Tremellen KP, Briggs NE, Dekker GA, Robertson SA. Seminal plasma pro-inflammatory cytokines interferon-gamma (IFNG) and C-X-C motif chemokine ligand 8 (CXCL8) fluctuate over time within men. *Hum Reprod* 2017 Jul 1;32(7):1373–1381.

30. Larsen MH, Bzorek M, Pass MB et al. Human leukocyte antigen-G in the male reproductive system and in seminal plasma. *Mol Hum Reprod* 2011;17:727–738.

31. Sharkey DJ, Glynn DJ, Schjenken, JE, Tremellen KP, Robertson SA. Interferon-gamma inhibits seminal plasma induction of colony stimulating factor 2 in mouse and human reproductive tract epithelial cells. *Biol Reprod* 2018; 99:514–526.

Chapter 18

Immunotherapy/IVIG, Prednisolone and Intralipid in IVF

Ole Bjarne Christiansen and Kathinka Marie Nyborg

18.1. Introduction

With the introduction of better ovarian stimulation protocols, improved embryo culture techniques and intracytoplasmatic sperm injection (ICSI), the vast majority of in vitro fertilization (IVF) and ICSI cycles will today end up with embryo transfer (ET). Despite transfer of seemingly good-quality embryos, recurrent implantation failure (RIF) may be the main reason that many couples will not succeed in having a child after several IVF/ICSI attempts. There is no consensus as regards the definition of RIF, but it usually includes a number of completed ET cycles (usually ≥ 3) and/or a cumulative number of morphologically good embryos transferred (usually ≥ 10) without the establishment of a successful pregnancy. Unfortunately, in many publications dealing with treatment of RIF it is not clear whether biochemical pregnancies and early miscarriages are included in the definition, which renders comparison of results difficult.

The causes of RIF are mainly undetermined and much disputed but genetic errors in the embryo definitively play a major role. Even morphological good embryos at the cleavage stage are often completely or mosaic aneuploid. Knowing the survival potential of such genetically abnormal embryos, it can be predicted that transferring them will in most cases result in non-implantation or pregnancy loss within a few days after implantation (= occult losses occurring before the possibility of detecting βhCG in the blood) but in some cases the transfer will probably result in biochemical pregnancy or clinical miscarriage [1].

In RPL after spontaneous conception, almost half of the clinical pregnancy losses are euploid with the frequency increasing with increased number of previous losses and decreased age of the woman. The substantial number of euploid losses emphasizes the important role for maternal factors in RPL, and there is no reason to believe that maternal risk factors for RPL will act differently in pregnancies conceived spontaneously or conceived after IVF/ICSI. Furthermore, there is no reason to believe that pregnancy losses due to maternal factors will not occur under a similar clinical picture as when the embryo is aneuploid: occult, biochemical and clinical losses.

Maternal risk factors for RPL and RIF theoretically comprise systemic or uterine disturbances of importance for early trophoblast attachment and invasion. Immune disturbances are main candidates as maternal risk factors for RPL/RIF being able to cause defect trophoblast invasion. Anti-phospholipid and anti-thyroid antibodies are more prevalent in both RPL and RIF patients than in controls and altered levels of peripheral blood natural killer (NK) cells and plasma or endometrial cytokines have been reported in both RPL and RIF patients [2,3]. Furthermore, the presence of specific maternal HLA-G polymorphisms seems to characterize both RPL and RIF patients [2]. None of these immune disturbances has per se been proven to be causative for RIF but are more likely to be markers for a general immune dysregulation in the women.

Believing that at least a proportion of RIF cases is associated with maternal immune disturbances, an obvious approach of treating these women is by immunotherapy. Various immunomodulatory interventions have been tested in randomized controlled trials (RCTs) in both RPL and RIF patients. Considering these disorders as overlapping entities, interventions that work in RPL are also suggested to work in RIF although with less efficiency since RIF may be a more heterogeneous condition than RPL. The majority and the highest-quality RCTs of immunotherapy have been performed in RPL, and only a minority in RIF patients. However, in this chapter the focus will be on immunotherapy for RIF. The focus will be on three kinds of immunotherapy: intravenous immunoglobulin (IvIg), glucocorticoids (prednisolone) and intravenous lipid emulsions (intralipid).

18.2 Intravenous Immunoglobulin

High-dose IvIg is an established treatment in many autoimmune and inflammatory diseases with a huge series of proven or suggested mechanisms of action. Some proven mechanisms of action in autoimmune diseases are: interaction with Fc-receptors, inhibition of cell adhesion, inhibition of formation of or elimination of immune complexes, interference with antigen presentation, effects on cytokines including neutralization of inflammatory cytokines and effects on apoptosis.

18.2.1 Intravenous Immunoglobulin – clinical Studies in RIF

IvIg has been tested in several RCTs in RPL patients with various results. However, a recent meta-analysis of all RCTs confirmed a significant therapeutic effect in patients with secondary RPL [4]. Several studies have evaluated IvIg treatment in infertile couples that failed to achieve a successful pregnancy after assisted reproductive techniques (ARTs) such as IVF/ICSI. In a first meta-analysis of three RCTs of IvIg treatment in patients with previous ART failures [5–7], a significant increase in the live birth rate (LBR) per woman was shown [8]. In the non-IvIg-treated groups, LBR was 19.3 per cent versus 36.0 per cent in the IvIg-treated group (p = 0.012).

The quality of the RCTs included in the meta-analysis was limited: in none of the trials, RIF was well defined especially whether the definition included biochemical losses and miscarriages after ART or only included ART attempts resulting in a negative βhCG test. Furthermore, there was lack of information about how allocation to IvIg or non-IvIg treatment was undertaken. In two trials, the reported outcome seemed to be cumulative outcome after several ART attempts. In one of the RCTs, only patients with anti-thyroid antibodies were included [6], whereas in the others, patients were not selected due to immunological biomarkers. Only one of the trials seemed to be a genuine placebo-controlled RCT [7].

In a study of 229 RIF patients published after this meta-analysis [9], IvIg infusion at the time of oocyte retrieval and in some patients during pregnancy seemed to result in higher LBRs after IVF compared to expected rates published in Canadian ART Registry 2010 (Table 18.1). In patients with ≥4 prior IVF failures, LBR in IvIg-treated patients was 33 per cent compared with 15.7 per cent (p = 0.001) in patients with a similar history

Table 18.1 Effect of intravenous immunoglobulin in patients with two studies of recurrent implantation failure after IVF/ICSI

	Virro et al. [9]		Nyborg et al. [11]
Characteristics	Total (N = 229)	≥4 IVF failures (N= 78)	N = 52
Age (mean years)	34.6	34.8	34.6
Mean no. IVF failures	3.3	5.2	5.5
Mean no. miscarriages	0.8	0.7	3.3
Mean no. embryo transferred	2.0	2.0	
Pregnancy rate	60.3%	51.3%	
Live birth rate	40.2%	33.3%	36.5%
Live birth rate/embryo	23.3%	16.6%	
Expected pregnancy rate		23.4%**	
Expected birth rate	30%*	15.7%**	

* Canadian ART Register 2010 data
** Meldrum et al. [10]

from a multicentre study [10]. In the study by Virro et al. [9], patients, with abnormal NK cell testing or cytokine ratios in peripheral blood were given additional IvIg infusions or anti-tumour necrosis factor-α therapy and many were also treated with heparin.

In another study without an untreated control group [11], 52 patients with ≥3 miscarriages/biochemical pregnancies after IVF/ICSI (mean of 5.5 previous failed IVF/ICSI treatments) were treated with a combination of IvIg at the time of ET and subsequent repeated infusions until pregnancy week 14, in addition to 10 mg prednisone daily from first cycle day until week 7 of pregnancy. The LBR in the first IVF/ICSI attempt with immunomodulation was 36.5 per cent and after cumulative immunomodulatory treatments, it was 61.5 per cent (Table 18.1). The LBR in the first treatment with immunomodulation was comparable to the results in the previous studies [8–10].

A recent systematic review and meta-analysis on IvIg treatment for RIF including 10 studies of RIF patients treated with either IvIg or placebo/nothing concluded that IvIg treatment was significantly associated with higher implantation rates, clinical pregnancy rates and LBRs than placebo [12]. However, the validity of this meta-analysis is questionable primarily due to the limited methodological quality of several of the included studies, and there was significant heterogeneity between outcomes in the studies, which in reality prohibits them from being combined in a meta-analysis. LBRs in the most relevant of the studies included in the Li et al. meta-analysis and corresponding rates in non-IvIg-treated RIF patients are depicted in Figure 18.1 [12].

In one study in the meta-analysis, some of the patients had RPL rather than RIF [13] but all patients were included. In some studies, many patients in addition to IvIg got prednisolone, Humira, lymphocyte immunization or heparin [9,14]. In most studies, no random allocation to IvIg or non-IvIg was undertaken [9, 13–15]. The authors of the meta-analysis

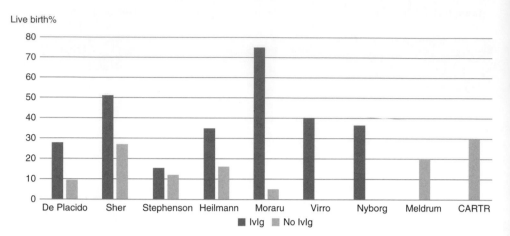

Figure 18.1 Live birth rates (LBRs) in patients with recurrent implantation failure after intravenous immunoglobulin (IvIg) treatment or no IvIg treatment in selected studies with or without internal controls.

In some of the studies, the depicted LBRs seem to be after the first IVF/ICSI attempt with IvIg (Stephenson et al. [7]; Virro et al. [9] and Nyborg et al. [11]), whereas in others, LBRs seem to represent cumulative outcome.

Expected LBRs after RIF in the background population are also depicted (Meldrum et al. [10], the Canadian ART Registry = CARTR)

classified several trials as 'placebo-controlled', although only one seemed to include a placebo-treated group [7].

Because of the limited validity of the Li et al. meta-analysis [12], conclusions of the efficacy of IvIg in RIF should in our view be based on the first meta-analysis, Clark et al. [8], which seemed to include only RCTs, and the only cohort study with a strict definition of RIF, treatment and outcome [11].

The Clark et al. meta-analysis [8] and the Nyborg et al. study [11] did very much agree that the LBR in RIF patients after IvIg (+/– prednisone) is 36 per cent, which appears to be a substantial improvement compared with the 15–23 per cent LBR reported in similar patients treated with placebo [7] or no IvIg [10].

18.2.2   Intravenous Immunoglobulin – shortcomings of Studies

The LBR in the IvIg-treated patients in the published studies exhibited very large variation ranging from 27.8 to 75 per cent, with the median LBR being 35 per cent (Figure 18.1). Potential methodological explanations for the huge variation in outcomes between studies are depicted in Figure 18.2.

The possible explanations for the variations are: (1) variation in the definition of RIF between the studies is a major factor; RIF patients who had never had a positive βhCG are by many clinicians considered to have a worse prognosis than those with repeated positive βhCGs, although this has never been adequately investigated in scientific studies; (2) random allocation to treatments in some studies but not in others; trials with random allocation between treatment/non-treatment have been documented to result in smaller treatment effects than non-randomized trials; (3) furthermore, it is important whether the outcome measure is outcome in the first subsequent pregnancy with immunotherapy or whether it is the cumulative outcome after several attempts of IVF/ICSI with immunotherapy; astonishingly, this very important information is not stated in several

Definition	Allocation	Outcome measure	Result of trial
RIF = ≥ 3 neg βhCGs after IVF	Adequate randomization	Live birth rate after first IVF	
			Small effect
RIF = ≥ 3 failed pregnancies after IVF	Adequate randomization	Live birth rate after first IVF	
			Moderate effect
RIF = ≥ 3 failed pregnancies after IVF	No randomization	Live birth rate after first IVF	
			Large effect
RIF = ≥ 3 failed pregnancies after IVF	No randomization	Cumulative birth rate after referral	
			Very large effect

Figure 18.2 Possible methodological variables of importance for the huge variation in the main outcome measure: live birth rate (LBR) between studies of immunotherapy (and other therapies) in recurrent implantation failure. Their predicted effect on recorded LBR in the studies is shown

publications. The very high LBR of 75 per cent in the study by Moraru et al. [13] is probably the outcome after IvIg treatments in consecutive ART attempts, although this is not completely clear.

Because of the aforementioned shortcomings in the relevant studies, it is for the time being not possible to conclude whether IvIg significantly improves the prognosis in RIF patients. Adequately randomized trials with clear definition of RIF and clear definition of the main outcome measure, preferably LBR in the first IVF/ICSI attempt with IvIg/placebo after referral, are urgently needed.

18.2.3 Intravenous Immunoglobulin Treatment – selection by Immune Biomarkers

Many advocates of the use of IvIg in RIF argue that the effect is largest in patients with immunological disturbances [14,16] since it is suggested to work by reducing harmful NK cell cytotoxicity or inflammatory cytokines [14]. Therefore, in many publications, the treatment has been targeted for patients with such disturbances: expanded NK cell populations [13–15], high Th1/Th2 ratios [14] or presence of thyroid antibodies [6](Table 18.2). The study by Nyborg et al. [11], however, did not find the treatment more efficient in patients with autoantibodies compared with those without. In many trials, RIF/RPL patients have been selected to IvIg therapy when peripheral blood CD56$^+$ NK cells > 12 per cent among all lymphocytes. However, CD56$^+$ NK cells > 12 per cent is a frequent finding (72 per cent in ICSI patients [17]) and the lack of validity of peripheral blood NK cell counts and many other biomarkers for identifying RIF patients with an immunological cause of RIF/RPL is highlighted in another chapter of this book. We believe that for the time being it is justified to include patients in RCTs of IvIg based exclusively on their well-characterized reproductive history rather than the presence of immunological biomarkers with uncertain importance.

Table 18.2 Characteristics of studies included in Figure 18.1

Study	Reproductive history	Selection due to immune biomarkers	Concomitant treatment
De Placido et al. [5]	≥3 unsuccessful ETs	No	No
Sher et al. [6]	No information	Positive for anti-thyroid antibodies	Heparin/low-dose aspirin
Stephenson et al. [7]	Repeated IVF failure	> 5% positive for anti-nuclear or anti-phospholipid antibodies	No
Heilmann et al. [15]	≥3 unsuccessful ETs	>12% CD56$^+$CD16$^+$ NK cells	Heparin in 2.7%
Moraru et al. [13]	Mean no. of 5.6 unsuccessful IVF attempts	Expanded number of NK or NKT-like cells in peripheral blood	No
Virro et al. 9]	≥2 IVF failures or unexplained infertility	Immune tests were used for deciding for additional immunotherapy	12% received additional immunotherapy and several got heparin
Nyborg et al. [11]	≥3 pregnancy failures after IVF/ICSI	No	10 mg prednisone

18.2.4 Intravenous Immunoglobulin – cost-effectiveness Analysis

Many clinicians have argued against the use of IvIg in RIF and RPL due to its high costs. The Danish pharmacies (without national health insurance coverage) charge approximately $5000 for three dosages of 25 g IvIg = 75 g, which reflect the amount of drug used in the majority of trials in one ART attempt with positive βhCG. If IvIg improves LBR from 20 to 35 per cent in an RIF patient (Figure 18.1) and one IVF treatment in Denmark costs approximately $4000, a cost-effectiveness analysis will probably show that the treatment is cost-effective. However, a valid cost-effectiveness analysis cannot be performed before more relevant RCTs have been carried out.

18.2.5 Intravenous Immunoglobulin – conclusion

Clearly, there is a need for good and large randomized, preferably placebo-controlled, trials of treatment with IvIg in patients with RIF. In these trials, RIF should be clearly defined and adequate doses of IvIg should be provided. Patients may be selected to the RCT due to presence of various biomarkers for immune dysfunction in order to identify a primary target group but the prevalence of these markers must be similar in the IvIg and placebo groups.

18.3 Prednisolone

Another kind of immunotherapy used in IVF/ICSI is glucocorticoid administration with, for example, prednisolone. Glucocorticoids have strong clinical effects in most autoimmune and inflammatory diseases and are widely used in clinical practice. It has been proposed that glucocorticoids may improve the intrauterine environment by reducing NK cell numbers, and suppress endometrial inflammatory cytokines [18]. Moreover, there is also some evidence the glucocorticoids may improve ovarian response in IVF/ICSI.

The use of glucocorticoids has been tested in two placebo-controlled trials in patients with RPL after spontaneous conception: one trial reported a 9 per cent higher LBR in patients getting high-dose prednisolone compared with placebo [19] and another smaller trial found a 20 per cent benefit [20]; however, in none of the trials was the treatment effect statistically significant.

18.3.1 Glucocorticoids in ART

No RCT of prednisolone has been performed in RIF patients but several trials have tested glucocorticoids, including prednisolone, in IVF/ICSI patients with no history of RIF. All trials where IVF/ICSI patients were randomized to periconceptional (mainly luteal phase) glucocorticoid treatment versus placebo or no glucocorticoids were included in a meta-analysis by Boomsma et al. [18]. In 13 trials, the authors found a borderline statistically significant increase in pregnancy rates after administration of glucocorticoids in IVF; odds ratio (OR) for pregnancy 1.50 (95 per cent CI 1.05–2.13) – whereas no significant effect was found in ICSI patients or in the whole group of IVF/ICSI patients; OR for pregnancy 1.15 (95 per cent CI 0.93–1.43). There were indications that glucocorticoids especially benefited IVF patients with a diagnosis of endometriosis. The authors of the meta-analysis made their conclusions with caution since the included trials were clinically very heterogeneous, few trials were blinded and drop-outs were poorly reported. In addition, only three trials reported on the main outcome measure: LBR, which was not significantly increased after glucocorticoids.

18.3.2 Glucocorticoids in RIF

The results of the aforementioned meta-analysis call for RCTs testing glucocorticoids in RIF patients; however, no such study has so far been performed. The cohort study by Nyborg et al. [11] tested the combination of IvIg to gestational week 14 and prednisolone to week 7 resulting in a subsequent high (36.5 per cent) LBR. The combination of IvIg and glucocorticoids is used in many autoimmune diseases and is believed to potentiate the effect compared with the effect of each drug. Therefore, testing the combined IvIg/glucocorticoid treatment in an RCT of RIF patients should be a priority in addition to testing glucocorticoids alone.

Unfortunately, due to their low costs, glucocorticoids, in contrast to IvIg, have already gained widespread use in clinical practice for treating RIF patients, but we and others consider this liberal use too premature.

In a recent article, Robertson et al. warn against uncritical use of glucocorticoids in ART [21]. The use of glucocorticoids to all RIF patients without selection is based on the assumption that abnormal immune activation is inconsistent with normal implantation and pregnancy. However, there is plenty of evidence that controlled inflammation and activation of the immune response are essential for embryo implantation; both these immune functions can be affected negatively by glucocorticoid administration. Therefore, in some instances, the treatment may be directly harmful and reduce implantation chance. Furthermore, prolonged prednisolone administration in pregnancy is associated with pre-term birth, diabetes and hypertension [19]. Robertson et al. argue that unless overt (auto) immune pathology is evident, utilization of glucocorticoids is not warranted [21]. The authors call for well-designed RCTs to define specific subgroups of RIF patients and diagnostic criteria that warrant glucocorticoid administration. We can only agree.

18.4 Intralipid

Intravenous lipid emulsions (such as intralipid) were initially developed to provide par-enteral nutrition. In recent years, intralipid has emerged as a treatment for poisoning by local anaesthetics and various other drugs.

It was initially reported that infusions of intralipid reduced the fetal resorption rate in specific mice matings. Roussev et al. reported that NK cell cytotoxicity declined after intralipid infusions to RIF patients to the same level as after IvIg infusions and extrapolated that intralipid had a beneficial effect in RPL [22]. Several other effects of intralipid on the immune function, which may play a role for implantation failure have been reported [23,24].

Due to the potential function on immune function and its much lower price compared with IvIg, intralipid is offered for the treatment of RPL and RIF in several clinics. Data on its effect in these reproductive disorders are, however, sparse and contradictive. One trial found that the LBR in RPL patients with intralipid treatment was similar (92 per cent) to that after IvIg (88 per cent) [25]. In another study, the LBR per treatment cycle in patients with a (poorly defined) history of reproductive failure and elevated NK cytotoxicity was 61 per cent in women treated with intralipid and 56 per cent for women treated with IvIg [24].

However, a recent small study [26] seriously questions the efficacy of intralipid in RIF. Among women aged 40–42 years with previous miscarriage or implantation failure, no clinical pregnancies occurred in patients receiving intralipid versus 30 per cent in untreated controls (p = 0.09). The authors concluded that peri-implantation intralipid infusions may actually be detrimental.

A series of serious adverse effects have been reported after the use of intravenous lipid emulsions, for example acute kidney injury, acute lung injury, venous thromboembolism, fat embolism, allergic reactions and increased susceptibility to infections. Good-quality RCTs of intralipid in well-defined patients with RIF younger than 40 years are therefore urgently needed.

18.5 Overall Conclusions

Cohort studies point to birth rates in RIF patients treated with IvIg, which are substantially higher than those reported in external control groups and RIF patients treated with peri-implantation IvIg can be promised a subsequent birth rate of approximately 35 per cent. However, only one small adequately placebo-controlled RCT on the topic has been con-ducted showing no or only a very small effect of IvIg in RIF. Adequately designed RCTs with clear definitions of RIF and the main outcome after treatment are urgently needed.

Periconception glucocorticoids seem to increase the chance of pregnancy in IVF patients but testing in RIF patients has not been done in RCTs. In theory, glucocorticoids may in some patients induce immune changes in the uterus that can reduce implantation chance, so until RCTs are done their use should be restricted to RIF patients with overt signs of autoimmunity.

In theory, the impact of intralipid on immune functions of significance for implantation is doubtful. The evidence for a positive clinical effect in RIF is completely absent, and it should not be used for treating RIF patients before testing in well-designed RCTs has been completed.

References

1. Macklon NS, Geraedts JP, Fauser BC. Conception to ongoing pregnancy: the 'black box' of early pregnancy loss. *Hum Reprod Update* 2002; **8**: 333–43.

2. Christiansen OB, Nielsen HS, Kolte AM. Future directions of failed implantation and recurrent miscarriage research. *Reprod BioMed Online* 2006; **13**: 71–83.

3. Sacks G, Yang Y, Gowen E et al. Detailed analysis of peripheral blood natural killer cells in women with repeated IVF failure. *Am J Reprod Immunol* 2012; **67**: 434–42.

4. Egerup P, Lindschou J Gluud C, Christiansen OB. ImmuREM IPD study group. The effects of intravenous immunoglobulins in women with recurrent miscarriages: A systematic review of randomized trials with meta-analyses and trial sequential analyses including individual patient data. *PLoS ONE* 2015: **10**: e141588.

5. De Placido G, Zullo F, Mollo A et al. Intravenous immunoglobulin (IVIG) in the prevention of implantation failure. *Ann N Y Acad Sci* 1994, **734**: 232–4.

6. Sher G, Maassarani G, Zouves C et al. The use of combined heparin/aspirin and immunoglobulin G therapy in the treatment of in vitro fertilization patients with antithyroid antibodies. *Am J Reprod Immunol* 1998; **39**: 223–4.

7. Stephenson MD, Fluker MR. Treatment of unexplained in vitro fertilization failures with intravenous immunoglobulins: A randomized, placebo-controlled Canadian trial. *Fertil Steril* 2000; **74**: 1108–13.

8. Clark DA, Coulam CB, Stricker RB. Is intravenous immunoglobulin (IVIG) efficacious in early pregnancy failure? A critical review and meta-analysis for patients who fail in vitro fertilization and embryo transfer (IVF). *J Assist Reprod Genet* 2006; **23**: 1–13.

9. Virro MR, Winger EE, Reed JL. Intravenous immunoglobulin for repeated IVF failure and unexplained infertility. *Am J Reprod immunol* 2012; **68**: 218–25.

10. Meldrum DR, Silverberg KM, Bustillo M, Stokes L. Success rate with repeated cycles of in vitro fertilization-embryo transfer. *Fertil Steril* 1998; **69**: 1005–9.

11. Nyborg KM, Kolte AM, Larsen EC, Christiansen OB. Immunomodulatory treatment with intravenous immunoglobulin and prednisone in patients with recurrent miscarriage and implantation failure after in vitro fertilization or intracytoplasmatic sperm injection. *Fertil Steril* 2014; **102**: 1650–5.

12. Li J, Chen Y, Liu C, Hu Y, Li L. Intravenous immunoglobulin treatment for repeated IVF/ICSI failure and unexplained infertility: A systematic review and a meta-analysis. *Am J Reprod Immunol* 2013; **70**: 434–47.

13. Moraru M, Carbone J, Alecsandru D, Castillo-Rama M et al. Intravenous immunoglobulin treatment increased live birth rate in a Spanish cohort of women with recurrent reproductive failure and expanded CD56$^+$ cells. *Am J Reprod Immunol* 2012; **68**: 75–84.

14. Winger EE, Reed JL, Ashoush S et al. Elevated preconception CD56$^+$16$^+$ and/or Th1: Th2levels predict benefit from IVIG therapy in subfertile women undergoing

IVF. *Am J Reprod Immunol* 2011; **66**: 394–403.

15. Heilmann L, Schorsch M, Hahn T. CD3-CD 56+CD16+ natural killer cells and improvement of pregnancy outcome in IVF/ ICSI failure after additional IvIg treatment. *Am J Reprod Immunol* 2010; **63**: 263–65.

16. Chernyshov VP, Dons´koi BV, Sudoma IO, Goncharova YO. Multiple immune deviations predictive for IVF failure as possible markers for IVIG therapy. *Immunol Letters* 2016; **176**: 44–50.

17. Coulam CB, Goodman C, Roussev RG, Thomason EJ, Beaman KD. Systemic CD56+ cells can predict pregnancy outcome. *Am J Reprod Immunol* 1995; **33**: 40–45.

18. Boomsma CM, Keay SD, Macklon NS. Peri-implantation glucocorticoid administration for assisted reproductive technology cycles. *Cochrane Database Syst Rev* 2012; **6**: CD005996.

19. Laskin CA, Bombardier C, Hannah ME et al. Prednisone and aspirin in women with autoantibodies and unexplained recurrent fetal loss. *New Eng J Med* 1997; **337**: 148–53.

20. Tang A-W, Alfirevic Z, Turner MA et al. A feasibility trial of screening women with idiopathic recurrent miscarriage for high uterine natural killer cell density and randomizing to prednisolone or placebo when pregnant. *Hum Reprod* 2013; **28**: 1743–52.

21. Robertson SA, Jin M, Yu D et al. Corticoid therapy in assisted reproduction-immune suppression is a faulty premise. *Hum Reprod* 2016; **31**: 2164–73.

22. Roussev RG, Acacio B, Ng SC, Coulam CB. Duration of intralipid's suppressive effect on NK cell's functional activity. *Am J Reprod immunol* 2008; **60**: 258–63.

23. Shreeve N, Sadek K. Intralipid therapy for recurrent implantation failure: new hope or false dawn? *J Reprod Immunol* 2012; **93**: 38–40.

24. Coulam CB, Acacio B. Does immunotherapy for treatment of reproductive failure enhance live births? *Am J Reprod Immunol* 2012; **67**: 296–303.

25. Meng L, Lin J, Chen L et al. Effectiveness and potential mechanisms of intralipid in treating recurrent spontaneous abortion. *Arch Gynecol Obstet* 2016; **294**: 29–39.

26. Check JH, Check DH. Intravenous intralipid therapy is not beneficial in having a live delivery in women aged 40–42 years with a previous history of miscarriage or failure to conceive despite embryo transfer undergoing in vitro fertilization-embryo transfer. *Clin Exp Obstet Gynecol* 2016; **43**: 14–5.

Chapter 19

The Role of Heparin and Aspirin to Aid Implantation

Tarique Salman and Luciano G. Nardo

19.1 Introduction

Despite all the advances in the field of assisted reproductive technology (ART) more cycles still fail than succeed, to the disappointment of the couple trying to conceive as well as the treating clinician.

Embryo implantation is a complex process of signalling and interaction between the embryos and the endometrium to allow adhesion, nidation, and then trophoblast invasion.

Even when transferring single euploid embryos, live birth rates are 40–60 per cent in randomized controlled trials (RCTs) and miscarriage rate almost 25 per cent, so other factors rather than chromosomal errors play a major role in failed implantation and miscarriages; one possible mechanism is activation of the coagulation system.

19.2 Heparin

Heparin is a polysulfated glycosaminoglycan that interacts with proteins containing positively charged amino acids [1]. Low molecular weight heparin (LMWH) is a depolymerised form of the unfractionated heparin and has similar action with increased bioavailability and half-life, so is given once a day.

Heparin and LMWH have been used for the management of recurrent miscarriages (RM) in women with antiphospholipid (APL) syndrome [2]. A review by Buckingham and Chamley found infertile women, and those with recurrent in vitro fertilization (IVF) implantation failure, have an increased incidence of APL (22 and 30 per cent, respectively) compared with a healthy, fertile population, (only 1–3 per cent) [3]. A more recent review failed to show such a high prevalence and also concluded that most studies used different tests/criteria for the diagnosis of APL making it harder to reach a conclusion [4].

In women with APL and other thrombophilias such as anticardiolipin antibodies, the antibodies bind to human trophoblast cells β2-glycoprotien leading to poor placentation [5]. It is also suggested that thrombophilia causes micro-thrombi at the implantation site causing defective trophoblast invasion and implantation failure [6].

Moreover, heparin has been shown to be effective in improving implantation rates without the presence of thrombophilia [7]. There is some evidence that heparin modulates endometrial receptivity and decidualization of endometrial stromal cells and improves implantation. Researchers have shown that heparin increases the production of insulin-like growth factor (IGF-1) and inhibits the production of insulin-like growth-factor-binding protein (IGFBP-1) [8], and these proteins play an important role in endometrial development and receptivity during the implantation window [9].However, different studies have given conflicting results about the efficacy of heparin or LMWH in improving pregnancy rates.

There are three meta-analyses that looked at the effect of heparin or LMWH in women having IVF treatment [10, 11 and 12]. Seshadri and colleagues (10) analysed five RCTs that had live birth rate (LBR) as primary outcome and found no significant difference between treatment and control group. They looked as well at clinical pregnancy rate (CPR) as secondary outcome, and in five RCTs there was a trend towards higher CPR in the treatment group but this did not reach statistical significance (PR 1.23, CI 0.97–1.57), while four observational studies showed significant improvement in CPR in the treatment group (PR 1.83, CI 1.04–3.23) p=0.04 [10].

Akhtar and colleagues[11] looked at five RCTs and one observational study and showed that heparin treatment determined a significant improvement in LBR, and CPR but after excluding the observational study and using sensitivity analysis with random effects model, the difference was insignificant but with a trend towards improvement in CPR [11].

Potdar and colleagues [12] looked at two RCTs and one quasi-RCT, looking at women with recurrent implantation failure (RIF) defined as three or more failed transfers. Statistical analysis (fixed effect forest plot) for the primary outcome set as LBR in women with ≥3 RIF showed significant improvement in LBR with LMWH in the intervention group (37/127: 29 per cent) versus the control group (19/118: 16 per cent), RR 1.79, 95 per cent CI 1.10–2.90, p= 0.02. Sensitivity analyses for women with ≥3 unexplained RIF showed a trend towards improvement in LBR with LMWH but it was not significant for the intervention group (27/85: 32 per cent) versus the control group (18/77: 23 per cent), RR 1.36, 95 per cent CI 0.82–2.26, p=0.24. They also looked at miscarriage rate and found significant reduction in miscarriage rate in all three studies for the treatment group. Subgroup analysis for women with unexplained RIF showed a non-significant trend in the reduction of miscarriage rate.

It is therefore plausible to conclude that there is no clear evidence of the effectiveness of heparin or LMWH in improving LBR or CPR in IVF or RIF, although there is a trend towards improved outcome but non-significant. There is also some reduction in miscarriages with the use of heparin/LMWH.

Consequently, the use of heparin or LMWH in IVF should not be routinely applied unless indicated clinically due to thrombosis risk or as part of research trials into that topic.

Similarly in women with APL going through IVF, there is not enough evidence for the routine use of heparin or LMWH just on the basis of diagnosis of APL (as shown in meta analytical pooling); thus, the conclusion is that APL positive women do not have reduced IVF success compared to negative controls [13].

The American Society for Reproductive Medicine does not recommend the use of heparin or LMWH in women who are positive for APL and who are having IVF treatment. Women who are positive for APL with history of RM should be offered low-dose aspirin and heparin/LMWH as there is strong evidence to support their use to improve outcome in future pregnancies [14].

From the above we can conclude that there is not enough data to recommend the administration of heparin or LMWH for unexplained RIF or RM without the diagnosis of thrombophilia unless as part of larger RCTs that are still needed.

More recently, researchers have been looking at selecting a cohort of patients that might benefit more from heparin therapy during ART treatment. The naturally occurring anticoagulant protein Annexin A5 (ANXA5) was found to be significantly reduced on the placental villous surfaces in women with APS. ANXA5 is highly expressed on the surface of the syncytiotrophoblast and is important for the integrity of the placenta acting as an anticoagulant protein blocking negatively charged phospholipids from the coagulation reactions, it is also postulated that ANXA5 is essential for the repair and maintenance of the syncytiotrophoblast apical membrane preventing coagulation.

Measurement of ANXA2 M2 haplotype can serve as a biomarker for the reduced ANXA5 and increased risk of adverse pregnancy outcome, pre-eclampsia and growth restriction. This group might potentially benefit from heparin treatment [15].

19.3 Safety

Adverse effects have been poorly reported in most studies but have included small numbers of women with bleeding and bruising. The use of LMWH is less likely to be associated with such problems and does not require close monitoring.

19.4 Aspirin

Aspirin is an anti-platelet aggregation agent that inhibits cyclo-oxygenase enzyme, preventing the synthesis of thromboxane. Daily use of low-dose aspirin induces a shift from thromboxane A2 towards prostacyclin enhancing vasodilatation and blood perfusion.

It has been used as a cardio-protective and has also been shown to reduce the risk of intrauterine growth restriction and pre-eclampsia [16]. This has led to interest in aspirin use to improve implantation in RIF and IVF.

Several studies have shown conflicting results; some used aspirin only while others combined aspirin with heparin. Some studies looked at RM with APS while others looked at unexplained RM and unexplained failed implantation in IVF.

An early Cochrane review looking at treatment for RM with APS found that the use of unfractionated heparin with aspirin significantly reduced miscarriage compared to aspirin alone. Interestingly, three trials examining the use of aspirin alone found no significant difference [17].

Another review was to determine the effect of low-dose aspirin on the likelihood of pregnancy in women undergoing IVF/ICSI [18]. It did not show any significant improvement in CPR or LBR when aspirin was used against placebo or no treatment, although one study found improvement in implantation rate in egg recipients but no significant improvement in CPR or LBR.

They concluded that there is not enough evidence to support prescribing low-dose aspirin for women going through IVF.

A more recent Cochrane review looked at 13 studies, 2,653 patients. The meta-analysis showed no evidence of significant difference or improvement in LBR, CPR or miscarriage rate with the use of low-dose aspirin over no treatment or placebo. They also concluded that there is not enough evidence to recommend the use of aspirin in IVF cycles to improve success rate [19]. One of the largest studies in this review did show some improvement in CPR of 17 per cent.

We can see from the data above that there is not enough evidence of a significant benefit from using aspirin in IVF. There are indeed concerns regarding its safety; aspirin use for longer times or higher dose can cause bleeding problems and gastric ulcer. We would therefore recommend that aspirin should not be used in IVF unless as part of large RCTs.

Aspirin and heparin are effective in reducing miscarriage rates in women with RM and APS but studies so far have failed to show similar benefits in cases of unexplained RM or the assisted reproduction field.

References

1. Linhardt RJ, Wang HM Ampofo SA. New methodologies in heparin structure analysis and the generation of LMW heparins. *Advances in Experimental Medicine and Biology* 1992;313:37–47.

2. Rai R, Cohen H, Dave M. et al. Randomised controlled trial of aspirin and aspirin plus heparin in pregnant women with recurrent miscarriage associated with phospholipids antibodies (or antiphospholipid antibodies). *Br Med J* 1997;314:253–257.

3. Buckingham KL, Chamley LW. A critical assessment of the role of antiphospholipid antibodies in infertility. *J Reprod Immunol* 2009;80:132–145.

4. Chighizola CB, De Jesus GR. Antiphospholipid antibodies and infertility. *Lupus* 2014;23:1232–1238.

5. Di Simone N, Meroni PL, de Papa N et al. Antiphospholipid antibodies affect trophoblast Gonadotrophins secretion and invasiveness by binding directly and through adhered beta2-glycoprotein I. *Arthritis & Rheumatism* 2000;43:140–150.

6. Azem F, Many A, Ben Ami I et al. Increased rates of thrombophilia in women with repeated IVF failures. *Human Reproduction* 2004;19:368–370.

7. Urman B, Ata B, Yakin K et al. Luteal phase empirical low molecular weight heparin administration in patients with failed ICSI embryo transfer cycles: a randomized open-labelled pilot trial. *Hum Reprod* 2009;24:1640–1647.

8. Fluhr H, Spratte J, Ehrhardt J et al. Heparin and low-molecular-weight heparins modulate the decidualization of human endometrial stromal cells. *Fertil Steril* 2010;93:2581–2587.

9. Wilcox AJ, Baird DD, Weinberg CR. Time of implantation of the conceptus and loss of pregnancy. *N Engl J Med* 1999;340:1796–99.

10. Seshadri S, Sunkara SK, Khalaf Y, El-Toukhy T, Hamoda H. Effect of heparin on the outcome of IVF treatment: a systematic review and meta-analysis. *Reproductive Biomedicine Online* 2012;25:572–584.

11. Akhtar MA, Sur S, Raine-Fenning N et al. Heparin for assisted reproduction. *Cochrane Database of Systematic Reviews* 2013;8:CD009452.

12. Potdar N, Gelbaya TA, Konje JC, Nardo LG. Adjunct low-molecular-weight-heparin to improve live birth rate after recurrent implantation failure: a systematic review and meta-analysis. *Human Reproduction Update* 2013;19:674–684.

13. Hornstein MD, Davis OK, Massey JB, Paulson RJ, Collins JA. Antiphospholipid antibodies and in vitro fertilization success. A meta analysis. *Fertil Steril* 2000;73:330–333.

14. RCOG green top guideline no. 17.

15. Fishel S, Baker D, Greer I. LMWH in IVF-biomarkers and benefits. *Thrombosis Research* 2017;151(suppl1):S65–S69.

16. Collaborative low dose aspirin study in pregnancy, collaborative group CLASP; a randomised trial of low dose aspirin for the prevention and treatment of pre-eclampsia among 9364 pregnant women. *Lancet* 1994;343:619–629.

17. Empson MB, Lassere M, Craig JC, Scott JR. *Cochrane database of systematic reviews* 2005;2:CD002859

18. Gelbaya TA, Kyrgiou M, Li TC, Stern C, Nardo LG. Low dose aspirin for in vitro fertilization: a systematic review and meta-analysis. *Hum Reprod Update.* 2007 Jul-Aug;13(4):357–64.

19. Siristatidis CS, Basios G, Pergialiotis V, Vogiatzi P. *Cochrane Database of Systematic Reviews* 2016;11:CD004832.

Chapter 20

Early Pregnancy Loss
Causes and Prevention

Shreeya Tewary and Jan J. Brosens

20.1 Introduction

Miscarriage, defined as loss of pregnancy before the fetus reaches viability, is the most common complication in pregnancy [1]. Approximately 15 per cent of pregnancies end in clinical miscarriage, and 25–50 per cent of women experience at least one sporadic miscarriage during their reproductive years. The number of miscarriages in the United Kingdom alone is estimated to be 200,000 per year. Most miscarriages are sporadic and occur before 12 weeks of gestation. They frequently involve numeric chromosome errors in the conceptus. Recurrent pregnancy loss (RPL) is viewed as a condition distinct from sporadic miscarriage. It is estimated that 5 per cent of women experience two consecutive miscarriages, and approximately 1 per cent suffer three or more consecutive miscarriages [1].

Miscarriage, whether spontaneous or recurrent, can be highly variable in its presentation. In recent years, attempts have been made to unify the terminology used to describe pregnancy loss prior to viability. For example, the ESHRE Early Pregnancy Special Interest Group emphasized the importance of distinguishing non-visualized pregnancy loss [i.e. biochemical pregnancy loss and pregnancy loss of unknown location (PUL)] and miscarriage [2]. The latter category encompasses intrauterine pregnancy losses, visualized by ultrasound, that can be subclassified into anembryonic- (i.e. empty sac), yolk sac-, embryonic- (< 10 weeks' gestation) and fetal- (≥ 10 weeks' gestation) loss. The reason for distinguishing embryonic from fetal demise is that organogenesis is completed by ten weeks. Further, prior to ten weeks, the growth and development of the conceptus is predominantly dependent on histotrophic nutrition provided by uterine glands. After ten weeks, the haemochorial placenta is established and increasingly perfused by circulating maternal blood.

There is as yet no consensus definition for RPL; clinical criteria range from two miscarriages, consecutive or not, to three consecutive miscarriages, including non-visualized pregnancy losses or not. For clarity, we define RPL here as three consecutive pregnancy losses, irrespective of the stage of development. By convention, 'RPL' and 'recurrent miscarriage' are clinical terms with pathological connotation, unlike sporadic miscarriage. However, it is important to appreciate that cumulative live birth rates (LBRs) are high in RPL patients, irrespective of medical intervention. For example, several randomized double-blind placebo control studies reported LBR of 65 per cent or more in RPL patients assigned to the placebo group [3]. In RPL, the incidence of euploid fetal loss increases with each additional miscarriage, whereas the likelihood of a future successful pregnancy gradually decreases [4]. These observations indicate that RPL is a graded disorder with the level of severity defined by the number of previous pregnancy losses. Nevertheless, even after five consecutive miscarriages, the likelihood of a live birth in a subsequent pregnancy remains in excess of 50 per cent [1].

20.2 Associated Risk Factors and Perceived Causation

The management of RPL is vexed with problems and tangible progress in improving outcome for affected couples has been at best modest in recent decades. The underlying reasons are complex. Historically, the clinical approach to miscarriages is rooted in the concept that the placenta is a vulnerable, immature organ, easily perturbed by a host of factors, which – outside pregnancy – have little or no ill health effects. Consequently, it has become standard practice to investigate RPL patients for a range of subclinical disorders, ranging from endocrine perturbations, uterine anomalies, latent infections, thrombophilias, immune disorders and lifestyle factors (Figure 20.1). Following on from this supposition, any perturbation detected upon screening is often uncritically assumed to be causal; hence, the widely promulgated but misleading concept that 50 per cent of RPL cases are 'explained' and 50 per cent 'unexplained'. A second popular paradigm of RPL is based on the paradoxic immunological relationship between mother and fetus. The Nobel laureate Sir Peter Brian Medawar was also the first to propose that survival of the allogeneic conceptus requires an evasive mechanism based on the concept of self-/non-self-recognition in classical transplantation biology [5]. This concept not only kick-started the field of reproductive immunology but also spawned a battery of largely non-validated immune tests for RPL.

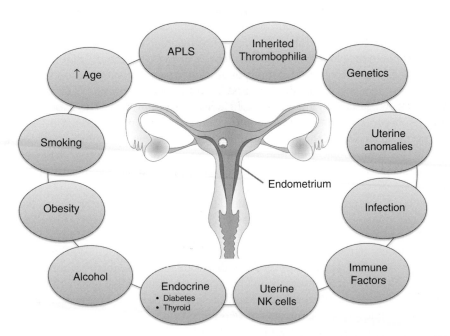

Figure 20.1 Factors perceived to cause recurrent pregnancy loss. Although many subclinical disorders and lifestyle factors are thought to converge onto the pregnant uterus, none are specific, meaning that they are also very prevalent in women with normal pregnancies. Increased maternal age is an important risk factor for aneuploid pregnancy loss, whereas obesity is associated with higher-order miscarriages in RPL patients

The dearth of convincing evidence for the pathological paradigms outlined above is clearly charted in a number of clinical guidelines from expert committees [6, 7]. A detailed discussion of all the evidence, or better lack thereof, is beyond the scope of this chapter. However, a number of general observations can be made. First, there is an abundance of cross-sectional studies in the literature, often small and underpowered, reporting putative risk factors that are more prevalent in RPL patients when compared to selected control subjects. For example, in excess of 100 susceptibility genes have been linked to RPL [8]. However, in most cases, the clinical significance of these polymorphisms on pregnancy outcome in RPL patients has not been tested in prospective cohort studies. The few polymorphisms that have been tested, such as ANXA5-1C/T, were found not to impact subsequent pregnancy outcome. Similarly, several studies have linked polycystic ovary syndrome (PCOS) to RPL, yet there is no evidence that PCOS increases the risk of further miscarriage in RPL subjects [8]. Second, there is the issue of biological plausibility, an essential component of the Bradford Hill criteria for disease causation. For example, based on modest associations in case-control studies, a dogged clinical concept is that inherent thrombophilias cause implantation failure and early miscarriage. However, prior to ten weeks, the conceptus develops in a hypoxic environment supported by histotrophic nutrition. In fact, histological analysis of maternal arterial connections with the intervillous space revealed that placental perfusion before the eighth week of pregnancy is improbable, which in turn renders it also unlikely that blood clots at the embryo-maternal interface are a genuine cause of miscarriages, at least not early pregnancy loss. Nevertheless, the incidence of Factor V Leiden (FVL) mutation, a prevalent inherited thrombophilia, is approximately 50 per cent higher in RPL patients but, importantly, its impact on subsequent outcome has not yet been established. This in turn leads to a third major issue: screening for subclinical disorders is only useful if subsequent treatment is effective in improving outcome for RPL patients. There has been no shortage of interventional studies. Our Pubmed search of randomized controlled trials (RCTs) and systematic reviews published in the last ten years yielded 142 studies reporting on drug interventions to prevent further miscarriage and improve life birth rate in RPL. A number of high-quality meta-analysis, systematic reviews and RCTs are summarized in Table 20.1. Overall, no clear or compelling strategy has emerged to prevent further miscarriages in RPL patients. Perhaps a notable exception is antiphospholipid syndrome (APS, also known as Hughes Syndrome), a systemic autoimmune disease defined by thrombosis and/or pregnancy morbidity in the presence of persistently positive antiphospholipid antibodies. A patient with APS must meet at least one of two clinical criteria (vascular thrombosis or complications of pregnancy) and at least one of two laboratory criteria including the persistent presence of lupus anticoagulant (LA), anticardiolipin antibodies (aCL) and/or anti-β2 glycoprotein I (anti-β2GPI) antibodies of IgG or IgM isotype at medium to high titres. Contrary to the widely held clinical view, overwhelming evidence has shown that pregnancy loss associated with APS is not primarily due to thrombotic events, but caused by decidual and placental inflammation [9].

It should be noted that the current RPL paradigms do not explain the high cumulative LBR in RPL nor can it account for the paradoxical association between RPL and superfertility. The term 'superfertility' is defined by an average monthly fecundity rate (MFR; i.e. the probability of achieving a pregnancy in one menstrual cycle) of >60 per cent. Normal MFR is approximately 20–30 per cent, whereas subfertility and infertility are defined by MFR of 1–5 per cent and 0 per cent, respectively. Based on time-to-pregnancy (TTP)

Table 20.1 Efficacy of medical intervention for the prevention of RPL

Intervention	Design	Author, Journal	Conclusion
Antiphospholipid antibody syndrome			
Pre- and post-conception LMWH + Aspirin vs. placebo	RCT	Ismail et al., *Int J Gynaecol Obstet.* 2016	No increase in LBR
UFH/LMWH + Aspirin vs. Aspirin alone	SR	Ziakas et al., *Obstet Gynecol.* 2010	UFH + Aspirin increases LBR
Aspirin/UFH/UFH + Aspirin/Prednisolone + Aspirin/IVIG + Aspirin	SR	Empson et al., *Cochrane.* 2005	Combined UFH and Aspirin may reduce pregnancy losses by 54%. Larger trials needed.
LMWH + Aspirin vs. IVIG	RCT	Triolo et al., *Arthritis Rheum.* 2004	LMWH + Aspirin increases LBR
Unexplained RPL			
IVIG	SR	Hutton et al., *BJOG,* 2007	No increase in LBR
	SR	Ata et al., *Fertil Steril.* 2011	
	RCT	Christansen et al., *BJOG,* 2015	
Progesterone	MA	Saccone et al, *Fertil Steril.* 2016	Inconclusive
LMWH + Folic acid vs. Folic acid alone	RCT	Shaaban et al. *Clin Appl Thromb Hemost.* 2016	Increase in LBR
LMWH vs. Placebo	RCT	Pasquier, *Blood.* 2015	No increase in LBR
LMWH vs. Multivitamins	RCT	Schleussner et al., *Ann Intern Med.* 2015	No increase in LBR
Aspirin/heparin/UFH	SR	De Jong PG et al, *Cochrane Database.* 2014	Inconclusive
Aspirin or LMWH	SR	Kaandorp et al., *Cochrane Database.* 2009	No increase in LBR
HCG	MA	Morley et al, *Cochrane Database.* 2013	No benefit
Lymphocyte Immunotherapy	SR	Cavalcante et al., *Arch Gynecol Obstet.* 2016	Inconclusive
GCSF vs. Placebo	RCT	Scarpellini et al, *Hum Reprod.* 2009	Inconclusive
Chinese Herbal Medicine	SR	Yang et al, *BMC Complement Altern* Med. 2013	Not recommended

Table 20.1 (cont.)

Intervention	Design	Author, Journal	Conclusion
Inherited Thrombophilia			
LMWH + Placebo vs. LMWH + Aspirin vs. Aspirin alone	RCT	Visser et al., *Thromb Haemost*. 2011	No increase in LBR

RCT: randomized controlled trial, SR: systematic review, MA: meta-analysis, LBR: live birth rate, UFH: unfractionated heparin, LMWH: low molecular weight heparin, IVIG; intravenous immunoglobulin, HCG: human chorionic gonadotrophin, GCSF: growth colony stimulating factor.

intervals, independent studies reported that 40 per cent of RPL patients are 'superfertile', which compares to the predicted incidence of 8 per cent. Interestingly, the incidence of superfertility is even higher in obese RPL patients [10].

20.3 Genomic Instability in Human Embryos

Although the clinical miscarriage rate is ~15 per cent, the incidence of preclinical attrition of implanted embryos is estimated to be 30–50 per cent. Intrinsic genomic instability of human embryos belies the exceptionally high attrition rate at implantation. Two decades of pre-implantation genetic research has unequivocally established that the majority – if not all – of human embryos harbour aneuploid blastomeres during early development. Chromosomal errors of meiotic origin in human embryos correlate strongly with maternal age, are biased towards maternal homologs and disproportionally affect smaller chromosomes (chromosomes 13, 15, 16, 18, 19, 21 and 22). By contrast, chaotic cell divisions caused by spindle abnormalities in early cleavage stage embryos result in complex mitotic aneuploidies that are independent of maternal age, frequently involve larger chromosomes, and are not biased towards either maternal or paternal homologs [11]. Some mitotic errors are catastrophic and cause developmental arrest prior to the blastocyst stage, thus contributing to the relatively low rate of human fertility. However, complex mosaic aneuploidies remain very prevalent in human blastocysts and many are compatible with a successful pregnancy outcome.

While numerous studies have investigated the incidence of aneuploidy in the early conceptus, little or no attention has been paid to the functional significance of aneuploid blastomeres in mosaic human embryos. The general assumption is that aneuploidy is a non-adaptive consequence of evolution, meaning that it is an erroneous by-product that conveys no reproductive advantages, only disadvantages. This concept may be fundamentally wrong. The purpose of reproduction is to ensure the survival of the species through change in the gene pool from generation to generation by such processes as mutation and natural selection. Different species employ different strategies to ensure reproductive success. For example, reproductive fitness in mice is based on quantity; characterized by rapid breeding cycles, multiple implantations, short gestation and large litter sizes. Selection in this species is arrived at mainly through intense sibling rivalry after birth. By contrast, human pregnancy requires prolonged investment in a single fetus at considerable cost to the mother. Intense selection following birth would be reproductively punitive and arguably imperil long-term survival of our species. Active selection of genetically diverse embryos at, or soon after, implantation seems a much more cogent strategy to ensure reproductive success.

It is important to emphasize that the reproductive blueprint of most species is not prescriptive but malleable. For example, while the incidence of chromosomal errors in pre-implantation murine embryos is very low, the developmental potential of experimentally induced mosaic embryos is not impaired as long as they also contain sufficient euploid cells [12]. On the other hand, transfer of a single embryo into a mouse foster mother almost always results in resorption, suggesting that reproductive boundaries are defined by cost-benefit considerations. Similarly, multiple pregnancies are not uncommon in humans but maternal cost and the risk of neonatal death increase sharply with each additional fetus.

20.4 Intrinsic and Extrinsic Embryo Selection

The incidence of aneuploidy in human embryos is estimated to be an order of magnitude higher than in other non-primate species. Some aneuploidies may cause embryonic demise prior to implantation, whereas others may have little detrimental impact on implantation or even promote invasion of the endometrium. For example, the single most common genetic aberration associated with clinical miscarriage is trisomy 16, a chromosome that contains several genes encoding for implantation-related serine proteases, including prostasin (PRSS8). Thus, to be reproductively successful, both intrinsic (i.e. embryonic) and extrinsic (i.e. uterine) mechanisms must operate to limit prolonged maternal investment in a failing pregnancy. Recent experimental studies have yielded no evidence that abnormal blasto-meres in mosaic embryos are preferentially sequestered in the trophoblast lineage. Instead, apoptosis appears to be the major mechanisms to eliminate genetically abnormal cells in the inner cell mass, which gives rise to the fetus proper. By contrast, cellular senescence has been identified as the primary mechanism to prevent expansion of abnormal trophectoderm cells, which form the placental interface between mother and offspring [12]. Cellular senescence is characterized by permanent cell cycle exit and secretion of matrix metalloproteinases and a host of inflammatory mediators, commonly referred to as senes-cence-associated secretory phenotype (SASP). This raises the possibility that aneuploid trophectoderm cells, like cancer cells, actively contribute to the invasiveness of the tropho-blast during the initial stages of the implantation process [5].

The human uterus has also evolved to minimize maternal investment in a failing pregnancy. The most salient sign of this evolutionary adaptation is menstruation. This remarkable phenomenon is triggered by falling progesterone levels in a handful of species, including Old World monkeys, that exhibit 'spontaneous' decidualization of the endome-trium, meaning that this process is initiated in response to maternal rather than embryonic cues. The coupling of spontaneous decidualization to menstrual shedding is nothing but an ingenious solution to deal with highly diverse and often chaotic human blastocysts: First, with cyclic tissue destruction being the default response in the human endometrium, an effective and safe 'disposal system' for aberrant but potentially highly invasive embryos is built into the cycle. Second, it also makes it incumbent on the implanting embryo to produce sufficient 'fitness' signals, such as human chorionic gonadotropin (hCG), to avoid inevitable rejection. Considering how indispensable this fitness signal is for embryo survival, it is not surprising that the human genome contains not one but six highly homologous *CGB* genes, coding for the beta polypeptide of hCG, which arose from multiple duplications of the ancestral *LHB* gene (coding for the luteinizing hormone beta polypeptide). Third, recent studies have shown that decidual cells are exquisite biosensors of embryo quality at implantation [13]. This is a critical point as active rejection at implantation results in preclinical attrition, whereas beyond this stage a clinical miscarriage ensues. To appreciate the role of an aberrant decidual process in RPL, a discussion of its physiological roles in pregnancy is warranted.

20.5 The Role of the Decidua in Early Pregnancy

20.5.1 The Decidual Pathway

Decidualization denotes the transformation of endometrial stromal cells into specialized secretory decidual cells that provide a nutritive and immune-privileged matrix essential for embryo implantation and placental development [5]. Decidualization is initiated during the mid-luteal phase of the cycle in response to elevated progesterone levels, paracrine signals and rising cellular cyclic adenosine monophosphate (cAMP) production. Typically, it commences with the transformation of stromal cells surrounding spiral arterioles during the mid-luteal phase of the cycle and then spreads to encompass the whole superficial endometrial layer as the cycle progresses. In parallel, the endometrium undergoes extensive remodelling effected by the influx of specialized immune cells, predominantly uterine natural killer cells and macrophages. At a molecular level, rising cellular cAMP levels activate the expression of decidua-specific transcription factors, such as CCAAT-enhancer-binding proteins (C/EBPs), Forkhead box protein O1 (FOXO1), Homeobox A10 (HOXA10) and HOXA11. Once the decidual process is initiated, the liganded progesterone receptor (PGR) physically binds decidua-specific transcription factors, thus maintaining and amplifying the expression of differentiation genes, including prolactin (PRL) and insulin-like growth factor-binding protein 1 (IGFBP1) [5].

Importantly, decidualization is not an on or off process but characterized by distinct functional phases (Figure 20.2). An early event in response to cAMP signalling in endometrial stromal cells is activation of NOX-4 (nicotinamide adenine dinucleotide phosphate oxidase-4), which triggers a burst of free radical production that kick-starts decidual gene expression. In parallel, decidualizing cells actively secrete a host of chemokines, interleukins and other inflammatory mediators, including alarmins such as interleukin (IL)-33, that are involved in innate immune cell activation. Feedback pathways ensure that the inflammatory decidual response is self-limiting, lasting between two and four days. Consequently, the initial decidual phase is followed by a profound anti-inflammatory response, characterized by simultaneous down-regulation of numerous chemokines and inflammatory mediators. In concert, continued progesterone signalling triggers massive up-regulation of 11β-hydroxysteroid dehydrogenase type 1 (11βHSD1), an enzyme that converts inert cortisone to active cortisol. This cortisol gradient in the decidua likely protects the invading allogeneic fetal trophoblast against a maternal immune response. Further, by silencing chemokine expression, decidual cells actively prevent effector T cells from entering the feto-maternal interface. The third and final phase involves the resolution of the decidual phenotype, triggered in a non-conception cycle by falling progesterone levels. During this phase, expression and secretion of inflammatory mediators by decidual cells rise again. This second inflammatory phase becomes irreversible upon recruitment and activation of various leukocyte populations (neutrophils, eosinophils, basophils, mast cells and macrophages) and results in tissue breakdown. Further, progesterone withdrawal also triggers

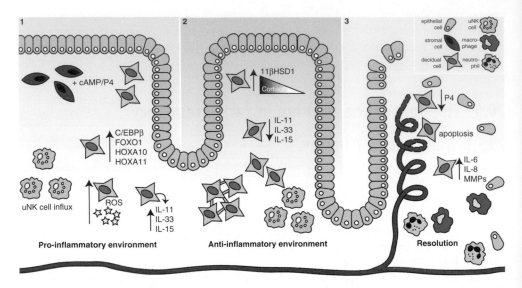

Figure 20.2 The decidual pathway. Distinct phases can be discerned upon decidual transformation of the endometrium. The first phase is characterized by an acute pro-inflammatory response that renders the endometrium transiently receptive to embryo implantation. The second phase is characterized by a profound anti-inflammatory response and the formation of a decidual matrix. Falling progesterone levels or functional progesterone withdrawal in pregnancy triggers a second inflammatory response, recruitment of various immune cells and tissue breakdown. P4: progesterone, cAMP: cyclic adenosine monophosphate, ROS: reactive oxygen species, MMPs: matrix metalloproteinases

a modest degree of apoptosis in decidual cells, which may well suffice to destabilize the terminal spiral arteries in vivo and initiate bleeding [5]. Thus, the term 'decidua', which is derived from the Latin verb 'decidere' (meaning to die, to fall off or to detach), truly captures the essence of the process.

20.5.2 Decidualization and the Window of Implantation

In recent years, new functions have been ascribed to each of the three phases of the decidual process, all of which are critical for a successful pregnancy outcome. First, the initial pro-inflammatory phase appears obligatory to transform the endometrium from a non-receptive to a receptive state. During this brief period, known as the 'window of implantation', the endometrium expresses an evolutionarily conserved repertoire of genes that enables a series of key events to take place, starting with the positioning of the embryo near the fundus of the uterus, absorption of uterine fluid, luminal 'closure' and apposition of the blastocyst on the endometrial surface epithelium. This is followed by stable adherence of the embryo to the apical surface of luminal epithelial cells, penetration through the luminal epithelium and its basal lamina and, finally, invasion of the stroma [5]. In humans, the receptive phenotype coincides with the mid-luteal phase (days 19–23) of a regular 28-day cycle. A limited implantation window is critical as it synchronizes two parallel but initially independent processes: embryo development and endometrial maturation. In polytocous species such as mice, a single endocrine signal not only functionally switches a progesterone-primed, pre-receptive endometrium to a receptive state but also activates the 'dormant' pre-implantation embryo. This obligatory maternal implantation signal consists of a transient rise in postovulatory oestradiol production, leading to increased uterine catechol oestrogen synthesis, which in turn renders the blastocyst competent for implantation. By contrast, there is no evidence that a distinct endocrine cue controls receptivity in the human endometrium, nor is there evidence that human embryos are capable of delaying implantation by entering a metabolically dormant state. Instead, the initial transient auto-inflammatory decidual response may have become the primary signal that drives receptivity in human endometrium. For example, when culture medium condition by human endometrial stromal cells is flushed through the mouse uterus, only the initial pro-inflammatory decidual secretome induces a receptive phenotype that allows implantation of transferred mouse blastocysts [14]. Furthermore, human blastocysts degrade when cultured in medium conditioned by undifferentiated endometrial stromal cells but not decidual cells, indicating that a non-receptive endometrium is actively embryotoxic.

20.5.3 Decidualization and Embryo Quality Control

The second decidual phase coincides with the embedding of the implanted embryo into the stroma. At this stage, the fully differentiated decidual cells, which are now tightly connected through gap and tight junctions, form a protective matrix around the early conceptus. Several mechanisms have been identified that renders the decidua exceptionally resistant to potentially harmful maternal inputs, including cessation of circadian gene oscillations, a huge increase in cellular free radical scavenging potential, selective silencing of stress-induced signalling through c-Jun N-terminal kinase (JNK) and p38 pathways, global cellular hypo-SUMOylation, and massive induction of phospholipase C-related catalytically inactive protein 1 (PRIP-1)[5, 15]. PRIP-1 is a progesterone-inducible scaffold protein that uncouples phospholipase C (PLC) activation downstream of Gq-protein-coupled receptors from intracellular Ca2+ release by attenuating inositol trisphosphate (IP3) signalling. The simultaneous silencing of all these pathways not only renders the decidua relatively autonomous but also ensures unimpeded progesterone signalling during the intense tissue remodelling in early pregnancy. Arguably, selective silencing of maternal inputs may also enhance the biosensor function of decidual cells by restricting signalling to embryonic cues [15].

The term 'biosensoring' was coined to describe the intrinsic ability of endometrial cells to respond to individual pre-implantation embryos in a manner that either supports further development or facilitates early rejection (Figure 20.3) [13]. Several in vitro models have highlighted the particular aptness of decidualizing cells in sensing poor-quality human embryos. In co-culture, human decidual cells respond to a developmentally impaired blastocyst by selectively down-regulating the secretion of multiple implantation factors. By contrast, undifferentiated endometrial stromal cells do not respond to a co-cultured embryo, irrespective of its quality. Furthermore, next-generation sequencing revealed a dramatic up-regulation of essential implantation and metabolic genes in murine uteri transiently exposed to the spent culture medium of developmentally competent human embryos. By contrast, exposure to the culture medium of low-quality human embryos triggers a stress response in the mouse uterus akin to the response observed in primary decidualizing human endometrial stromal cells [13]. Collectively, these in vivo and in vitro studies suggest that the embryo is subjected to both positive and negative selection pressures at implantation. The mechanism that imparts responsiveness of decidual cells to poor-

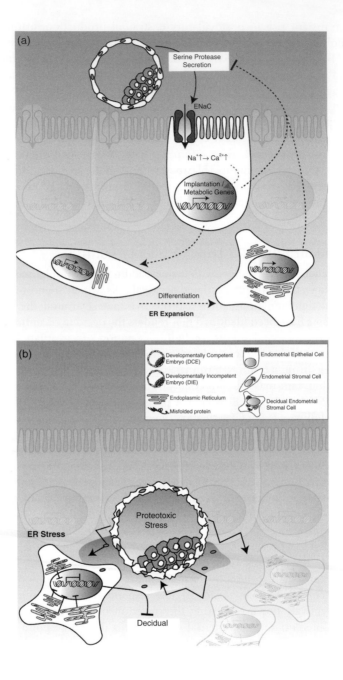

Figure 20.3 Positive and negative embryo selection at implantation. A. Serine proteases produced by developmentally competent embryos elicit calcium (Ca2+) signalling in endometrial cells through cleavage of epithelial sodium channels (ENaC), leading to expression of implantation and metabolic genes that are essential for post-implantation embryo development. B. By contrast, metabolic overdrive and proteotoxic stress in developmentally incompetent embryos that have breached the luminal endometrial epithelium trigger an endoplasmic reticulum (ER) in surrounding decidual cells, which in turn induces a hostile microenvironment that promotes early rejection

quality human embryos is not well defined. Microarray analysis identified HSPA8 as the most dysregulated decidual gene out of 450 genes responsive to signals from developmentally impaired human embryos. HSPA8 encodes heat shock 70 kDa protein 8 (HSC70), a key regulator of cellular protein homeostasis. HSC70 levels increase upon decidualization in parallel with expansion of the endoplasmic reticulum that drives the secretory phenotype of differentiating stromal cells. Hence, the importance of this molecular chaperone increases as decidualizing cells expand their secretory machinery, which may explain why undifferentiated stromal cells are not bequeathed with a biosensor function [13].

20.5.4 Decidualization and Endometrial Plasticity

The resolution phase of the decidual process is equally important for reproductive success. Menstruation, which virtually always precedes pregnancy, is thought to be an example of physiological preconditioning that prepares uterine tissue for the vascular remodelling and hyper-inflammation associated with deep haemochorial placentation. In most tissues, injury is a potent cue for activation of resident adult stem and progenitor cells that mediate repair. Not surprisingly, the cycling human endometrium is rich in mesenchymal stem cells (MSC), which reside in a specialized niche around the spiral arteries in both the basal and superficial layers. Human endometrial MSC (eMSC) are multipotent and capable of forming endometrial stroma when injected under the kidney capsule of immunocompromised mice. They express specific cell surface markers, such as Sushi Domain containing 2 (SUSD2) or co-expression of CD146 and platelet-derived growth factor receptor beta (PDGFRβ) [16]. Transcriptomic analysis demonstrated that eMSC first give rise to a more committed but still clonogenic population of cells before differentiating into mature stromal fibroblasts. Menstruation is followed by rapid oestrogen-dependent growth of the endometrium during the proliferative phase of the cycle. Consequently, the stromal compartment of the endometrium consists of a community of resident cells, ranging from eMSC, activated progenitor cells to mature and senescent cells. Iterative cycles of tissue destruction and repair are arguably essential for homeostatic balancing of the various subpopulations of stromal cells that, collectively, determine the quality of the decidual response. It also follows that the cycling human endometrium is intrinsically dynamic, meaning that the decidual response may not only vary from cycle to cycle but even recalibrate in response to miscarriage [17].

20.6 Aberrant Decidualization and RPL

Aberrant decidual responses in purified primary endometrial stromal cell cultures have been linked to a variety of reproductive disorders, including endometriosis, PCOS, and recurrent miscarriage [17]. These groundbreaking studies demonstrated that the responsiveness of endometrial cells to steroid signals and other cues is not predetermined but occurs in a disease-specific manner. The hallmark of the endometrium in RPL is a disordered and prolonged pro-inflammatory decidual response. This excessive initial inflammatory decidual response in turn prolongs the 'window of receptivity', promotes out-of-phase implantation, and disables embryo selection. Consequently, poor-quality embryos are not disposed of in a timely manner and high-quality embryos implant in an unsupportive environment. Both scenarios lead to clinical miscarriage. Further, lack of quality control at implantation is clinically reflected as 'superfertility', which is commonly reported by many RPL patients.

Immunoprecipitation of methylated DNA coupled to sequencing revealed that primary endometrial stromal cells isolated from RPL patients lack a genome-wide epigenetic signature associated with pluripotent cells. This signature, defined by DNA methylation at specific motifs in CA-rich loci, is lost in most somatic cells but becomes re-established upon reprogramming into pluripotent stem cells [18]. The association between RPL with eMSC deficiency was further validated by measuring the colony-forming unit-fibroblast activity of freshly isolated endometrial stromal cells from mid-luteal biopsies. Furthermore, the level of depletion of eMSC correlates with the severity of RPL phenotype as defined by the number of previous miscarriages. Lack of epigenetic stemness features in cultured stromal cells was further associated with intragenic hypomethylation and reduced expression of *HMGB2*. High Mobility Group Box 2 (HMGB2) is a multifaceted protein involved in chromatin bending and DNA damage repair. It was also identified as a major co-activator of the PGR. In endometrial stromal cells, knockdown of HMGB2 leads to cell cycle exit, activation of the DNA damage repair pathway, cellular senescence and an impaired decidual response. Taken together, these data indicate that RPL is associated with loss of endometrial plasticity, defined by stem cell deficiency, heightened cellular senescence and limited differentiation potential [18].

20.7 Clinical Perspective

Disease paradigms matter in medicine. A wrong paradigm inevitably leads to futile investigations and ineffective treatments. The search over many decades for subclinical disorders that explain RPL has yielded little supportive evidence, nor has it resulted in preventative strategies that actually work. The discovery of intrinsic genetic instability in human embryos combined with the emerging concept of active uterine selection provides a new ontological dimension to early pregnancy loss; and the ramifications are potentially far-reaching. For example, the discovery of specific endometrial defects associated with RPL, such as eMSC deficiency, opens up the possibility of pre-pregnancy screening of women at risk of miscarriage. This strategy, however, will require a more in-depth understanding of the mechanisms that control endometrial homeostasis from cycle to cycle. Put differently, it is equally essential to understand the mechanisms that enable a successful pregnancy to occur after multiple failures as it is to define the primary causes of RPL. While the role of decidualizing endometrial stromal cells in RPL is increasingly understood, defects in other cellular endometrial compartments, including the glandular epithelial cells, are as yet poorly defined. One major obstacle has been the inability to propagate primary endometrial epithelial cells efficiently in culture, especially when isolated from secretory endometrium. However, a new technique that enables establishment of adult stem cell-derived endometrial glandular organoids promises to overcome this pertinent hurdle [19].

If the fate of a conceptus is determined at implantation, treatments initiated in pregnancy are likely to be ineffective, a conjecture increasingly supported by disappointing results of numerous interventional clinical trials (Table 20.1). Instead, the therapeutic focus should be on optimizing the endometrium before implantation and pilot studies aimed at boosting eMSC in RPL patients are ongoing. The design of clinical trials also needs re-evaluation as many miscarriages are 'inevitable', for example when caused by chromosomal errors. Cumulative LBRs in RPL patients would be a more sensible approach to measure the effectiveness of medical intervention. Finally, there is a need for increased awareness of the psychological morbidity associated with early pregnancy loss. Miscarriage, and especially RPL, is unique in encompassing both a bereavement and personal clinical pathology. A new narrative around miscarriage, grounded in its biological context, may well help couples to come to terms with their loss.

Acknowledgement

We thank Drs Joanne Muter and Emma Lucas for their assistance in preparing this chapter.

References

1. Rai R, Regan L. Recurrent miscarriage. *Lancet* 2006;**368**:601–611.

2. Kolte AM, Bernardi LA, Christiansen OB et al. Eshre special interest group EP. Terminology for pregnancy loss prior to viability: a consensus statement from the ESHRE early pregnancy special interest group. *Hum Reprod* 2015;**30**:495–498.

3. Coomarasamy A, Williams H, Truchanowicz E et al. A Randomized trial of progesterone in women with recurrent miscarriages. *N Engl J Med* 2015;**373**:2141–2148.

4. Ogasawara M, Aoki K, Okada S, Suzumori K. Embryonic karyotype of abortuses in relation to the number of previous miscarriages. *Fertil Steril* 2000;**73**:300–304.

5. Gellersen B, Brosens JJ. Cyclic decidualization of the human endometrium in reproductive health and failure. *Endocr Rev* 2014;**35**:851–905.

6. Practice Committee of the American Society for Reproductive M. Evaluation and treatment of recurrent pregnancy loss: a committee opinion. *Fertil Steril* 2012;**98**:1103–1111.

7. The Investigation and Treatment of Couples with recurrent First-trimester and Second-trimester Miscarriage. Green-top Guideline No. 17. Royal College of Obstetrics & Gynaecology, April 2011.

8. Sugiura-Ogasawara M. Recurrent pregnancy loss and obesity. *Best Pract Res Clin Obstet Gynaecol* 2015;**29**:489–497.

9. Pantham P, Abrahams VM, Chamley LW. The role of anti-phospholipid antibodies in autoimmune reproductive failure. *Reproduction* 2016;**151**:R79–90.

10. Bhandari HM, Tan BK, Quenby S. Superfertility is more prevalent in obese women with recurrent early pregnancy miscarriage. *BJOG* 2016;**123**:217–222.

11. McCoy RC, Demko ZP, Ryan A et al. Evidence of Selection against Complex Mitotic Origin Aneuploidy during Preimplantation Development. *PLoS Genet* 2015;**11**:e1005601.

12. Bolton H, Graham SJ, Van der Aa N et al. Mouse model of chromosome mosaicism reveals lineage-specific depletion of aneuploid cells and normal developmental potential. *Nat Commun* 2016;**7**:11165.

13. Brosens JJ, Salker MS, Teklenburg G et al. Uterine selection of human embryos at implantation. *Sci Rep* 2014;**4**:3894.

14. Salker MS, Nautiyal J, Steel JH et al. Disordered IL-33/ST2 activation in decidualizing stromal cells prolongs uterine receptivity in women with recurrent pregnancy loss. *PLoS One* 2012;**7**: e52252.

15. Muter J, Brighton PJ, Lucas ES et al. Progesterone-Dependent Induction of

Phospholipase C-Related Catalytically Inactive Protein 1 (PRIP-1) in Decidualizing Human Endometrial Stromal Cells. *Endocrinology* 2016;**157**:2883–2893.

16. Gargett CE, Schwab KE, Deane JA. Endometrial stem/progenitor cells: the first 10 years. *Hum Reprod Update* 2016;**22**:137–163.

17. Lucas ES, Dyer NP, Fishwick K, Ott S, Brosens JJ. Success after failure: the role of endometrial stem cells in recurrent miscarriage. *Reproduction* 2016;**152**: R159–166.

18. Lucas ES, Dyer NP, Murakami K et al. Loss of Endometrial Plasticity in Recurrent Pregnancy Loss. *Stem Cells* 2016;**34**:346–356.

19. Turco MY, Gardner L, Hughes J et al. Long-term, hormone-responsive organoid cultures of human endometrium in a chemically defined medium. *Nat Cell Biol* 2017;**19**:568–577.

Is the Endometrium in Women with PCOS Compromised?

Terhi T. Piltonen

21.1 PCOS Endometrium and ART

Even though women with polycystic ovary syndrome (PCOS) are as likely to get at least one child as the general population [1], the diagnosis remains as the most common reason for anovulatory infertility; thus, these women are overrepresented among women undergoing assisted reproductive technologies (ART). Although anovulation can be solved in many cases with ovulation induction medication, the metabolic component remains often unsolved in ART contributing to subfertility in these women. Besides ovarian dysfunction there are several studies showing that the endometrial function is also compromised in women with PCOS, mostly related to anovulation. However, studies have also implied that even with ovulation, the endometrial function in women with PCOS remains unoptimal [2,3]. Indeed, there are several clinical manifestations that imply endometrial dysfunction in PCOS. The first reported endometrium-related clinically adverse outcome was miscarriage risk that was suggested to be increased in women with PCOS [4], even independently of body mass index (BMI) and ART [5], although not all studies agree [1]. Furthermore, affected women have been shown to present with a three- to fourfold increased risk for pregnancy-induced hypertension and preeclampsia, and a twofold higher chance of premature delivery [6,31].

The most crucial health burden for PCOS endometrium is the abnormal and unfavorable metabolic state and obesity in these women that also increases the need for ART. In addition to the impaired oocyte quality and the need for higher doses of gonadotrophins in in vitro fertilization (IVF), it is likely that adverse metabolic phenotype (women presenting with amenorrhea, hyperandrogenism, obesity, diabetes, hypertension) also affects the preconceptional endometrial milieu in women with PCOS [7]. In fact, some adverse outcomes may be derived from abnormal trophoblast invasion and placentation in cases of PCOS shown as altered placental histology with increased inflammation, thrombosis, and poor placental development even in uncomplicated PCOS pregnancies [8]. As for clinical practice, several studies have been evaluating the optimal treatment protocol for women with PCOS for ART. Recently, aromatase inhibitors were shown to yield higher live birth rates (LBRs) in women with PCOS compared with clomiphene citrate, possibly partly due to more beneficial implantation profile [9]. Indeed, a recent study reported secretory-phase endometrial gene expression profile more favorable for implantation in women using letrozol compared with clomiphene citrate [10]. Also, IVF protocol plays a role. For women with PCOS being in high risk for ovarian hyperstimulation syndrome (OHSS), antagonist protocol is recommended. However, despite the antagonist protocol, a high number of oocytes are still commonly retrieved, causing high levels of estrogen and

Table 21.1 Different endometrial markers in proliferative phase, in secretory phase, and in hyperplasia in women with PCOS

Marker	PE	SE	
Glucose metabolism			
IGFBP-1		▼	SE (in vitro) ▼ (Piltonen 2015)
GLUT 4	▼		PE▼, HP▼ (Li 2015); PE▼ (Fornes 2010); Zhai PE▼ (Zhai 2012*); PE▼ (Ujvari 2014*)
IRS-1	▼		PE▼ (Fornes 2010); PE▼ (Ujvari 2014*)
Glucose action	▼		PE▼ (Kim 2010*); PE▼ (Piltonen 2013*)
Inflammation			
TNFR1/TNFR2		△	△(Orostica 2016)
NfKb		△	△(Orostica 2016)
IL-6	△	△	PE△ (Piltonen 2013*); SE (in vitro)△ (Piltonen 2015)
CCL2 (MCP-1)	△		PE △(Piltonen 2013*)
IL-8	△	△	PE△ (Piltonen 2013*); SE (in vitro)△ (Piltonen 2015)
RANTES		△	SE (in vitro)△ (Piltonen 2015)
uNK-cells		▼	SE▼(Matteo 2010*)
Macrophages		△	△(Orostica 2016)
MMPs			
MMP2		△	SE (in vitro)△ (Piltonen 2015)
MMP3		△	SE (in vitro)△ (Piltonen 2015)
Steroid hormone action			
HOXA10		▼	SE▼(Taylor JCEM), downregulated in EC (ref)
AR	△	△	PE(-) (Piltonen 2013*); SE △ (Quezada 2006 FS*); PE△, HP△ (Li 2015); HP△(Villavicencio 2006)
PR		△	SE △(Margarit 2010*)
Era	△(-)	△	PE(-) (Piltonen 2013*); PE(-) (Kim 2010*); SE△(Gregory 2002)
			PE?△ and HP△(Villavicencio 2006); SE△(Quezada 2006 FS*); SE△(Margarit 2010*)
Erb	△	(-)	SE (-) (Quezada 2006 FS*); PE?△ and HP△(Villavicencio 2006)
(avb3) integrin	▼	▼	PE▼ (Kim 2010*); SE▼(Quezada 2006 FS*); ▼progestin treatment (Lopez 2014)
MUC1		△▼	SE△ovulatory PCOS, ▼anovulatory PCOS (Margarit 2010*)
Steroid horomone co activators			
AIBI	△	△	PE?△(Villavicencio 2006); SE△(Gregory 2002)
TIF2		△	SE△(Gregory 2002)
NCoR	(-)		PE?(-)(Villavicencio 2006)

PE, proliferative phase; SE, secretory phase; HP, hyperplasia
▼, decreased; △, increased; (-), no difference
*BMI-matched controls/no difference in BMI compared with controls
Modified from Piltonen T.T. "Polycystic ovary syndrome: Endometrial markers." Best Pract Res Clin Obstet Gynaecol. 2016

Table 21.2 Altered endometrial function in women with PCOS undergoing ART

Endometrial distress	Metabolic burden	Hyperandrogenism	ART
Strategies	Weight control/ reduction	Weight control/ reduction	Preferably Letrozol in OI vs. CC
	Exercise	Metformin	Preferably priming with progestin vs. OCPs
	Metformin		Avoiding OHSS (antagonist, GnRH-a trigger)
			Combining Metformin with ART early enough
			Freeze all?

progesterone in these cycles possibly having unfavorable effects on endometrial milieu and implantation. In fact, increased numbers of oocytes (>20) retrieved in IVF was recently associated with preterm birth and low birth weight suggesting altered placentation possibly related to ovarian hyperstimulation that provokes unhealthy hormonal and inflammatory environment [11].

Besides optimizing ovulation induction and IVF stimulation, it is important to study the PCOS endometrium characteristics also outside the context of ART. The most common endometrial abnormalities in women with PCOS are presented (Table 21.1) as well as the current efforts to improve endometrial implantation in these women (Table 21.2).

21.2 Endometrial Abnormalities in Women with PCOS

During the past years, an increasing number of studies have revealed several endometrial characteristics/markers related to the PCOS phenotype possibly explaining some of the unfavorable endometrium-related clinical manifestations. Owing to the heterogeneous nature of the PCOS population, it is possible that some of the findings may only be manifest in the most severe cases as the metabolic effects of obesity, hyperinsulinemia, and inflammation, for example, are difficult to separate from the syndrome itself. Unfortunately, limited number of studies have reported or taken into consideration the effects of obesity in their study setup or when interpreting the results. This should be, however, noted when evaluating the effect of PCOS per se [2].

21.2.1 Steroid Hormone Receptors

Anovulatory women with PCOS experience a chronic progesterone-deficient state in their endometrium because of absence of corpora lutea. As progesterone should knock down estrogen effect in secretory-phase endometrium by downregulating estrogen receptors (ERs), anovulation leads to chronic estrogen exposure and continuous mitogenic distress. Indeed, persistent ER/ERα expression in glandular epithelium and/or stroma is the most well-characterized endometrial abnormality in women with PCOS [2], although some studies that have included women with PCOS and controls with similar BMI do not agree. This may imply that different phenotypes may exist or that increased proliferation is specifically linked to obesity. Supporting the prolonged estrogen effect, the women with PCOS have been reported to present with an increased proliferation (upregulation of mitogen-inducible gene 6, cyclin B1 and cyclin E2) in clomiphene citrate – or progesterone-induced secretory-phase endometrium [2]. Interestingly, also, increased expression of p160 steroid receptor coactivator expression has been shown to be increased in PCOS endometrium possibly facilitating ERα activation and modulating estrogenic effects. Recent data also suggest that altered ratio of ERa/ERb might relate to impaired endometrial phenotype [2].

Besides anovulation-related progesterone deficiency in PCOS endometrium, recent studies have also suggested endometrial progesterone resistance in these women [12]. Several genes related to progesterone effects in human endometrium and implantation like *HOXA10*, integrin, claudin-4 and mucin-1 (MUC1) expression have been shown to be blunted in spontaneous or clomiphene citrate-induced secretory-phase PCOS endometrium. Furthermore, similarly to ER, alterations in the progesterone receptor alpha (PRα) and β isoform ratio have also been suggested to modulate steroid hormone action in human endometrium. Indeed, a recent clinical trial showed altered secretory-phase PRa/b expression in women with PCOS. Moreover, decidualization, a progesterone-driven mandatory event for successful implantation, has been shown to be compromised in PCOS. A recent in vitro study reported blunted decidualization response (with an altered inflammatory profile) of endometrial stromal cells in a subset of women with PCOS, showing a decreasing trend in PR expression simultaneously with reduced expression of decidualization marker insulin-like growth facto-binding protein-1 (IGFBP-1) compared with decidualized samples [12]. As decidualized endometrial stromal cells seem to have an active role in embryo selection [13], impaired decidualization capacity in these cells may result in impaired embryo selection potential.

PCOS endometrium has increased androgen receptor (AR) expression that may relate to low progesterone levels or blunted progesterone action [2]. As for reproduction, no correlations between early miscarriage and serum T levels or increased risk of pregnancy complications particularly related to hyperandrogenism have been found, despite in vitro finding of reduced *HOXA10* expression in connection with T and DHT. Assessing the isolated role of hyperandrogenism in endometrial function is challenging in PCOS, as hyperinsulinemia promotes hyperandrogenism in ovarian theca cells, thus androgens and insulin have simultaneous direct effects on endometrial functions. Interestingly, lowering androgen levels with combined contraceptives prior to IVF has not been found to improve live birth rates (LBRs) in women with PCOS [32]. Combined contraceptives induced impairment in glucose tolerance and increased systemic insulin levels may complicate the conclusions. Further research is needed to investigate whether androgen actions via ARs independently promote endometrial abnormalities in cases of PCOS, offering possible therapeutic approaches prior IVF.

21.2.2 IGF, IGFBP-1, and GLUT-4

Insulin resistance and systemic hyperinsulinemia are common findings in both lean and obese women with PCOS and genes related to insulin signaling have been shown to be altered in the endometrium in women with PCOS [3]. Insulin signals via the insulin receptors (IRs) and IGF receptors (IGFRs), which are upregulated in secretory-phase endometrium and involved in the peri-implantation period in feto-maternal crosstalk. The IGF-I and -II systems are also linked to insulin action and involved in the implantation process, and the IGF-binding ability of IGFBP-1 balances the effect of IGFs in the endometrium [3]. Balanced insulin action controls trophoblast invasion and placentation as insulin has been shown to reduce/inhibit endometrial decidualization and *IGFBP-1* in stromal fibroblasts [33]. The restricting effect of insulin on *IGFBP-1* can be reversed by using inhibitors of insulin signaling. Indeed, hyperinsulinemia may promote shallow trophoblast invasion, possibly explaining the increased risks for conditions related to poor placentation like pregnancy-induced hypertension and preeclampsia in women with type-2 diabetes or PCOS [6]. To support this, a recent study by Chang and colleagues showed decreased implantation, clinical pregnancy, and ongoing pregnancy rates among insulin-resistant women with PCOS, compared with noninsulin-resistant PCOS women, even after controlling for age, BMI and lipid levels [14].

Besides endometrial IGFBP-1 regulation, insulin also controls for glucose uptake in cells, which is facilitated by glucose transporters (GLUTs). Furthermore, insulin alone acts as a potent growth factor and stimulates androgen synthesis in ovarian theca cells, promoting hyperandrogenism. Insulin also worsens hyperandrogenism by decreasing sex hormone-binding globulin (SHBG) and IGFBP-1 synthesis in the liver, leaving more biologically active T, E2, and IGF in the circulation. The results of recent studies suggest that testosterone (T) alone may promote insulin resistance in human endometrial stromal fibroblasts and reduce expression of IR-1 and GLUT4 in endometrial epithelial cells, raising the question of whether there is an altered endometrial insulin signaling and insulin resistance especially in hyperandrogenic women with PCOS. Indeed, abrupt changes in insulin signaling with altered IR and/or GLUT4 expression have been reported in the endometrium in women with PCOS; however, it has been related to hyperinsulinemia rather than hyperandrogenism, although these often coexist in PCOS. In any case, metabolic derangements impair endometrial health and function in women with PCOS, probably increasing the risks of pregnancy complications if present during the periconceptional period warranting common guidelines and recommendation for metabolically compromised women with PCOS going through ART.

21.2.3 Inflammation and Immune Cells in PCOS Endometrium

The endometrium harbors various resident and transient immune cells that together with a unique cytokine and chemokine environment play a central role in normal endometrial function [15,16]. The inflammatory and immune cell profiles fluctuate in response to hormonal changes during the menstrual cycle, with the follicular phase having T-cell dominance and the secretory phase showing increased numbers of macrophages and especially uterine natural killer cells (uNK cells). Increased numbers of peripheral NK cells (CD56+) and decreased numbers of uNK cells have been found in women experiencing recurrent miscarriage, although clinical application regarding uNk cell characterization in women still awaits further studies.

The cytokine/chemokine secretion is also regulated by hormonal fluctuations and the cytokines most likely serve as endometrial homing signal for systemic stem cell recruitment and endometrial regeneration [16]. Moreover, cytokines are also key factors orchestrating implantation. For example, leukemia inhibitory factor (LIF), interleukins (IL) 1, 6, 11, and 15, and chemokine (C-C motif) ligands (CCLs) 2, 4, 5, 8, and 14 increase toward the mid-secretory phase [15] suggesting a role in embryo guidance; thus, balanced cytokine secretion profile is mandatory for initiation of healthy pregnancy. Indeed, an altered endometrial inflammatory stress response toward trophoblast invasion may compromise pregnancy.

A study with endometrial biopsy samples from the mid-secretory phase of nonpregnant women reported lower levels of IL-6 in women with previous recurrent miscarriage. Interestingly, recently women with PCOS were reported to present with an altered endometrial inflammatory profile with compromised cytokine secretion characteristics [17,18]. Furthermore, another study reported a subset of PCOS eSFs with an abnormal progesterone response also presenting increased inflammation compared with decidualized samples from controls or women with PCOS with normal decidualization response [12]. Whether these women would also be at a higher risk for impaired implantation, recurrent miscarriage or pregnancy complications remain to be determined.

21.4 Optimizing Endometrial Health in Women with PCOS Undergoing ART

21.4.1 Lifestyle

Obesity being a common factor in PCOS, lifestyle interventions are recommended as the first-line therapy prior to ART. In fact, a modest weight reduction of 5–10 percent has been suggested to be efficient to improve fertility [19,20,34]. Unfortunately, lifestyle programs have shown only modest long-term outcomes; thus, medical and surgical therapy is often needed especially in women with morbid obesity [20]. A recent randomized controlled trial (RCT), however, could show benefit of lifestyle intervention on reproductive outcome compared with oral contraception priming only. On average, 6 kg weight loss could improve ovulation rate, although no difference was observed in clinical pregnancy rate (CPR) or LBR [21]. In a smaller randomized study, a lifestyle intervention with diet and exercise was also shown to improve menstrual cycle and endometrial glucose metabolism and steroid hormone receptor profile suggesting beneficial effect on endometrial function [22].

Smoking is one of the major players impairing endometrial function and oocyte quality in women impairing the IVF success at least by 30 percent. Some studies have suggested PCOS women being more often smokers compared with other women, possibly related to weight-controlling efforts; thus, lifestyle advice is needed also in this area.

21.4.2 Hormonal Treatment and ART

Given that hyperandrogenism has been suggested as an independent factor for subfertility, a recent study investigated the effect of continuous oral contraceptive use for 16 weeks prior to conception (natural or through ART) compared with progestin only regimens. Despite lowering serum testosterone, the OC use was associated with lower CPR and LBR after fresh embryo transfer (ET) compared with progestin priming [21]. As the mechanism of these medications differ as for their effect on ovarian function it is possible that the difference is explained by their pituitary control and high affinity of ethinyl estradiol (EE) on ERs. Pituitary down-regulation might be prolonged affecting luteinizing hormone/follicle-stimulating hormone (LH/FSH) secretion possibly also carrying their effects on subsequent cycles in cases of only partial recovery. EE with high affinity to ERs perhaps may also have prolonged down-regulatory effect on PRs in the endometrial cells. The progestins, on the other hand, in most cases have only local endometrial and cervical effects without pituitary effects. However, in cases of PCOS endometrial shedding prior ART may not be beneficial at all [23].

As mentioned in the beginning of this chapter, aromatase inhibitor Letrozol was shown to have better outcomes in ovulation induction (OI) as for LBR compared with clomiphene in a previous RCT [9]. No difference was found in the pregnancy loss between the groups, although letrozol resulted in thicker endometrium compared with clomiphene that has shown to have selective antagonist effect on endometrium in some patients. Due to OHSS risk in PCOS, antagonist protocol is recommended with agonist trigger and "freeze only" strategy. Interestingly, a recent study showed that "freeze only" policy in noncomplicated PCOS pregnancies results in higher LBR and reduced miscarriage rate, although there was increased preeclampsia rate related to frozen embryo transfer (FET) cycles [24]. As for FET cycles, in a large dataset with non-PCOS segregation of the data, the OI cycles seemed to be as successful as the hormone replacement therapy cycles for ET [25].

Interestingly, a recent study showed tamoxifen, a selective estrogen receptor modulator (SERM) as potential therapy for thin endometrium especially in women with PCOS [35]. Tamoxifen was able to increase endometrial thickness from 6mm to 9mm resulting in decrease in cycle cancellation and higher CPR as well as LBR per transfer compared with natural/hormonal or OI cycles. The result implies that some patients with thin endometrium may benefit from tamoxifen pretreatment after failing with other endometrium preparing medications/natural cycle prior FET treatments, however further studies are warranted. In any case Letrozol seems to perform better than clomiphen and should be the first choice if available for usage.

21.4.3 Metformin

Metformin is widely used in women with PCOS; however, the results regarding its usefulness to improve LBR in ART or natural cycles are still somewhat under debate. Even though metformin has been shown to improve menstrual cycle regularity, by itself metformin is not as effective as OI medication in inducing ovulation [34]. In previous RCT, metformin combined with clomiphene in OI protocol failed to improve LBR, although the women were quite obese in this study [26]. Another RCT from Norway, which randomized pregnant women with PCOS (58 percent spontaneous pregnancies) to use metformin starting from 5 to 12 gestational week onward until the delivery, also failed to show benefits from metformin use [27]. A Finnish study, on the other hand, randomized women with PCOS undergoing ART to use metformin already three months prior ART initiation until gestational week 12, and was able to show increased LBR especially in obese women with PCOS [28]. This result was supported by a recent Cochrane Review and WHO guideline indicating metformin-improving LBR when combined with gonadotrophin-induced ovulation induction [20,29]. Although metformin might be able to reduce the risk for OHSS, it also seems to increase weight gain in offspring, although the results are preliminary. Further studies related to offspring health are warranted.

21.4.4 "Freeze only" Strategy

During IVF cycles, the high estrogen and progesterone concentrations may desynchronize implantation window and thus likely alter the endometrial milieu. In women with PCOS, hCG, commonly used to trigger ovulation during IVF, results in excessive steroid hormone response for up to five days as shown in our previous studies [30]. IVF-related altered endometrial environment is also supported by studies showing that 30 percent of the women with good prognosis and a euploid single blastocyst embryo do not achieve pregnancy. Thus, fresh ET, especially in cases with high oocyte count, may not be an optimal choice. Indeed, some studies have suggested that "freeze only" policy might improve pregnancy outcomes in IVF even outside OHSS cases. In fact, a recent publication showed improved LBR in women with PCOS chosen for elective embryo cryopreservation and FET program compared with PCOS women with fresh ET (49.3 percent vs. 42 percent) [24]. Interestingly, the FET cycles also had 10 percent lower pregnancy loss rate compared with fresh ETs. Antagonist protocol was used in all cycles and all OHSS cases were excluded. Surprisingly though, "freeze only" protocol resulted in higher preeclampsia rate (4.4 percent vs. 1.4 percent) implying that not all adverse outcomes related to IVF and high steroid hormone concentrations are solved with "freeze all" strategy.

21.5 Summary

There is emerging evidence that the endometrium in women with PCOS is compromised. Some of the abnormalities are related to obesity and ART and some to PCOS per se. Even though ART is being offered in cases of infertility, there are also several lifestyle and medical approaches that have been shown to improve endometrial function. As for ART, common clinical guidelines and protocols should be followed to guarantee safety and optimal outcome in cases of PCOS. Future studies assessing ART-related treatment outcomes, preferably LBR, but also pregnancy outcomes and offspring health are warranted.

References

(1) West S, Vahasarja M, Bloigu A et al. The impact of self-reported oligo-amenorrhea and hirsutism on fertility and lifetime reproductive success: results from the Northern Finland Birth Cohort 1966. Hum Reprod 2014;29:628–633.

(2) Piltonen TT. Polycystic ovary syndrome: Endometrial markers. Best Pract Res Clin Obstet Gynaecol 2016; 37:66–79.

(3) Giudice LC. Endometrium in PCOS: Implantation and predisposition to endocrine CA. Best Pract Res Clin Endocrinol Metab 2006;20:235–244.

(4) Joham AE, Boyle JA, Ranasinha S, Zoungas S, Teede HJ. Contraception use and pregnancy outcomes in women with polycystic ovary syndrome: data from the Australian Longitudinal Study on Women's Health. Hum Reprod 2014;29:802–808.

(5) Palomba S, Falbo A, Russo T et al. Pregnancy in women with polycystic ovary syndrome: the effect of different phenotypes and features on obstetric and neonatal outcomes. Fertil Steril 2010;94:1805–1811.

(6) Palomba S, de Wilde MA, Falbo A et al. Pregnancy complications in women with polycystic ovary syndrome. Hum Reprod Update 2015;21:575–592.

(7) Doherty DA, Newnham JP, Bower C, Hart R. Implications of polycystic ovary syndrome for pregnancy and for the health of offspring. Obstet Gynecol 2015;125:1397–1406.

(8) Koster MP, de Wilde MA, Veltman-Verhulst SM et al. Placental characteristics in women with polycystic ovary syndrome. Hum Reprod 2015;30:2829–2837.

(9) Legro RS, Brzyski RG, Diamond MP et al. Letrozole versus clomiphene for infertility in the polycystic ovary syndrome. N Engl J Med 2014;;371:119–129.

(10) Wallace KL, Johnson V, Sopelak V, Hines R. Clomiphene citrate versus letrozole: molecular analysis of the endometrium in women with polycystic ovary syndrome. Fertil Steril 2011;96:1051–1056.

(11) Sunkara SK, La Marca A, Seed PT, Khalaf Y. Increased risk of preterm birth and low birthweight with very high

number of oocytes following IVF: an analysis of 65 868 singleton live birth outcomes. Hum Reprod 2015;30:1473–1480.

(12) Piltonen TT, Chen JC, Khatun M et al. Endometrial stromal fibroblasts from women with polycystic ovary syndrome have impaired progesterone-mediated decidualization, aberrant cytokine profiles and promote enhanced immune cell migration in vitro. Hum Reprod 2015;30:1203–1215.

(13) Brosens JJ, Salker MS, Teklenburg G et al. Uterine selection of human embryos at implantation. Sci Rep 2014;4:3894.

(14) Chang EM, Han JE, Seok HH et al. Insulin resistance does not affect early embryo development but lowers implantation rate in in vitro maturation-in vitro fertilization-embryo transfer cycle. Clin Endocrinol (Oxf) 2013;79:93–99.

(15) Maybin JA, Critchley HO, Jabbour HN. Inflammatory pathways in endometrial disorders. Mol Cell Endocrinol 2011;335:42–51.

(16) Khatun M, Sorjamaa A, Kangasniemi M et al. Niche matters: The comparison between bone marrow stem cells and endometrial stem cells and stromal fibroblasts reveal distinct migration and cytokine profiles in response to inflammatory stimulus. PLoS One 2017 April 18;12(4):e0175986.

(17) Matteo M, Serviddio G, Massenzio F et al. Reduced percentage of natural killer cells associated with impaired cytokine network in the secretory endometrium of infertile women with polycystic ovary syndrome. Fertil Steril 2010;94:2222–2227.

(18) Piltonen TT, Chen J, Erikson DW et al. Mesenchymal stem/progenitors and other endometrial cell types from women with polycystic ovary syndrome (PCOS) display inflammatory and oncogenic potential. J Clin Endocrinol Metab 2013;98:3765–3775.

(19) Meldrum DR. Introduction: Obesity and reproduction. Fertil Steril 2017;107:831–832.

(20) Balen AH, Morley LC, Misso M et al. The management of anovulatory infertility in women with polycystic ovary syndrome: an analysis of the evidence to support the development of global WHO guidance. Hum Reprod Update 2016;22:687–708.

(21) Legro RS, Dodson WC, Kris-Etherton PM et al. Randomized Controlled Trial of Preconception Interventions in Infertile Women With Polycystic Ovary Syndrome. J Clin Endocrinol Metab 2015;100:4048–4058.

(22) Hulchiy M, Nybacka A, Sahlin L, Hirschberg AL. Endometrial Expression of Estrogen Receptors and the Androgen Receptor in Women With Polycystic Ovary Syndrome: A Lifestyle Intervention Study. J Clin Endocrinol Metab 2016;101:561–571.

(23) Diamond MP, Kruger M, Santoro N et al. Endometrial shedding effect on conception and live birth in women with polycystic ovary syndrome. Obstet Gynecol 2012;119:902–908.

(24) Chen ZJ, Shi Y, Sun Y et al. Fresh versus Frozen Embryos for Infertility in the Polycystic Ovary Syndrome. N Engl J Med 2016;375:523–533.

(25) Groenewoud ER, Cohlen BJ, Al-Oraiby A et al. A randomized controlled, non-inferiority trial of modified natural versus artificial cycle for cryo-thawed embryo transfer. Hum Reprod 2016;31:1483–1492.

(26) Legro RS. Metformin as adjuvant therapy to IVF in women with PCOS: when is intention-to-treat unintentional? Hum Reprod 2011;26:2043–2044.

(27) Vanky E, Stridsklev S, Heimstad R et al. Metformin versus placebo from first trimester to delivery in polycystic ovary syndrome: a randomized, controlled multicenter study. J Clin Endocrinol Metab 2010;95:E448–55.

(28) Morin-Papunen L, Rantala AS, Unkila-Kallio L et al. Metformin improves pregnancy and live-birth rates in women with polycystic ovary syndrome (PCOS): a multicenter, double-blind,

placebo-controlled randomized trial. J Clin Endocrinol Metab 2012;97:1492–1500.

(29) Bordewijk EM, Nahuis M, Costello MF et al. Metformin during ovulation induction with gonadotrophins followed by timed intercourse or intrauterine insemination for subfertility associated with polycystic ovary syndrome. Cochrane Database Syst Rev 2017 January 24;1:CD009090.

(30) Piltonen T, Koivunen R, Perheentupa A et al. Ovarian age-related responsiveness to human chorionic gonadotropin in women with polycystic ovary syndrome. J Clin Endocrinol Metab 2004;89:3769–3775.

(31) Hsu JY, James KE, Bormann CL et al. Mullerian-inhibiting substance/anti-Mullerian hormone as a predictor of preterm birth in polycystic ovary syndrome. J Clin Endocrinol Metab 2018 Sep.

(32) Legro, RS, Dodson WC, Kris-Etherton PM et al. Randomized Controlled Trial of Preconception Interventions in Infertile Women With Polycystic Ovary Syndrome. J Clin Endocrinol Metab 2015 Nov;100 (11):4048–58. doi: 10.1210/jc.2015-2778. Epub 2015 Sep 24.

(33) Ujvari, D, Jakson I, Babayeva S et al. Dysregulation of In Vitro Decidualization of Human Endometrial Stromal Cells by Insulin via Transcriptional Inhibition of Forkhead Box Protein O1. PLoS One 2017 Jan 30;12(1):e0171004. doi: 10.1371/journal.pone.0171004. eCollection 2017.

(34) Teede HJ, Misso ML, Costello MF et al. Recommendations from the international evidence-based guideline for the assessment and management of polycystic ovary syndrome. Hum Reprod 2018.

(35) Ke H, Jiang J, Xia M et al. The Effect of Tamoxifen on Thin Endometrium in Patients Undergoing Frozen-Thawed Embryo Transfer. Reprod Sci 2018 Jun 25;6:861–866. doi: 10.1177/1933719117698580. Epub 2017 Mar 27.

Index